HEALTHY BY DESIGN

Building and Remodeling Solutions
for Creating Healthy Homes

Healthy
by Design

*Building and Remodeling
Solutions for Creating
Healthy Homes*

D A V I D   R O U S S E A U
J A M E S   W A S L E Y

Hartley & Marks
PUBLISHERS

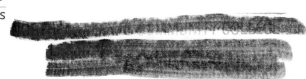

Published by

HARTLEY & MARKS PUBLISHERS INC.
P. O. Box 147   3661 West Broadway
Point Roberts, WA   Vancouver, BC
98281   V6R 2B8

LIBRARY OF CONGRESS CATALOGING-IN-PUBLICATION DATA
Rousseau, David.
    Healthy by design : building and remodeling solutions for creating healthy
homes / by David Rousseau, James Wasley.
        p.   cm.
    Includes index.
    ISBN 0-88179-135-0
    1. Interior decoration—Health aspects. I. Title.
NK2113.R68   1996
613.5—dc20   96-34085
                                                                         CIP

Design and composition by The Typeworks
Cover design by Diane McIntosh

Set in SCALA and SCALA SANS

Printed in the U.S.A.

CONTENTS

ACKNOWLEDGMENTS

First, thanks to Vic Marks and all of the staff at Hartley & Marks for still believing in books, and for motivating me to write, even when I don't have time for it.

Thanks also to co-author James Wasley, my healthy-building colleague, for his insight, contributions and commentary. Because he came into the project after it was underway, his contributions to the book far outweigh the time he was allotted to prepare them.

Thanks to Rick Fedoruk for his prompt and precise graphic production, and for usually knowing exactly what was meant by a few hasty sketches and notes on a fax page.

Thanks also to my family, friends and some of my clients who patiently tolerated neglect while I was consumed in finishing this book.

And special thanks to Susan Juby, editor, whose considerable talents, perseverance and organizational ability kept the forest in view when the rest of us were lost in the trees.

—DAVID ROUSSEAU, SEPTEMBER 1997

INTRODUCTION

When we try to pick out anything by itself, we find that it is bound fast by a thousand invisible cords that cannot be broken to everything in the universe... —JOHN MUIR, *JOURNAL*, 27 JULY 1869

Everything is connected to everything else. This maxim of ecology is the touchstone for our values and work as architects and authors. In *Healthy By Design* we focus on the importance of personal health, as illustrated in the case studies, and provide information for designing, buying, building and renovating living spaces for personal health, but this book goes beyond designing strictly for personal health. Though we have limited our scope to housing, we have introduced some variety in the building types discussed. We have introduced examples representing a wide range of climates, site conditions and design approaches, each with distinctively different requirements for healthy design. Since the problems of unhealthy housing are often specific design and construction pitfalls that can be avoided or solved, we discuss technical details that make a building "healthy by design."

If the "green" environmental movement that John Muir helped to found has anything to offer, it is the conviction that personal health is not separable from the health of the planet. This is the driving idea behind much of the creative problem solving that is loosely defined as "green" design. From our perspective, a discussion of healthy house design always leads to discussions of all sorts of other environmental concerns, from land use patterns to landfill capacity, to energy efficiency, acid rain and rain forest preservation. The challenge is to grapple with interconnections, not only within the realm of healthy building design, but also between health and other social and environmental concerns. We define health, resource conservation and energy efficiency as a spectrum of concern and attempt to place each case study within the spectrum. Our goal is promote solutions to the problems of health and energy efficiency, resource conservation, affordability and beauty. This harmonizing of competing factors is not only "green" design, it is also "good design," and it depends, in part, on an understanding of the evolution of the housing industry over the last half of the 20th century.

Construction technology, materials, and mechanical systems have changed dramatically over the last 50 years, and many of the problems and possibilities that this book addresses are related to those developments. Construction materials in particular changed radically as a result of the chemical revolution that followed the Second World War. Suddenly, synthetic materials were everywhere, promising less maintenance and longer product life. They offered new esthetic potential and were inexpensive. They even promised a healthier future, and delivered one to the extent that household surfaces became easier to clean. New mechanical equipment such as furnaces and air conditioners meant that fuel sources were cleaner and combined temperature and humidity control became possible.

While many petrochemical-based products later turned out to have toxic effects, these negatives were not immediately apparent. Environmentalism in its modern form did not come to the construction industry until the energy crises of the mid-1970s. At that point, rapidly rising energy costs made a strong case for conservation and reinforced the more general argument of the environmental movement that consumption equaled pollution. Buildings were identified as major consumers, wasting energy and creating pollution by their poor heating and cooling performance. Interest in energy efficient houses quickly spread. During this time, three trends developed: climate-responsive design was reinvigorated; mechanical equipment began to compete on the basis of efficiency; and increased levels of insulation coupled with airtight construction became the norm.

Tighter construction gained the most acceptance of these three trends. Site-responsive design required too much care, and better mechanical equipment too much capital, but insulation was easy for builders to add and did not change the visual appearance of the home. Insulation and weatherproofing in some older houses could also be inexpensively retrofitted, a self-help strategy that was widely promoted. The amount of energy saved as a result of such conservation measures outpaced most analysts' expectations, producing energy surpluses far more economically than new energy production could hope to. These gains made possible many important environmental victories, such as the creation of the Arctic National Wildlife Refuge, because it could be shown that oil drilling in that fragile ecosystem was not necessary with the success of the new conservation movement.

Unfortunately, the first generation of superinsulated houses also exposed the flaws of the innovations with which they were built. Sealing houses as tightly as thermos bottles had several disastrous consequences.

First, it amplified the unhealthy chemical soup that modern interiors had become due to the introduction of synthetic materials and household products. Second, it produced a wave of experimentation with even more toxic, high-performance insulation products, such as urea formaldehyde. Third, it created unanticipated potential for moisture to attack both the building and its occupants. Some houses built in the late 1970s were completely destroyed by rot within a decade, and many people developed health problems from exposure to high levels of mold, as well as to formaldehyde and a long list of other chemicals. By the early 1980s sick building syndrome was a familiar household concept for many and "healthy housing" was becoming a new priority.

As concern faded about energy supply, it became painfully clear that pollution was the next serious crisis facing the modern world. The earth's ability to absorb the wastes of industrialization seemed increasingly limited, and while the environmental legislation of the 1970s had targeted large industrial sources of air and water pollution, individual consumers were still producing mountains of garbage, much of it indestructible or toxic. States sued each other for access to landfills, and trash barges wandered the seas, unwelcome in any port. The construction industry was again singled out as a major contributor to the crisis, and the move to recycling building materials and to using recycled products in new construction took off.

And so we have begun to close the ecological loop, seeing buildings as holding devices for materials that are constantly in motion but never discarded, and working toward reducing both the energy input and the pollution outflow of what we build. This change in philosophy is apparent in many of the new composite products which are specifically formulated to be nontoxic. And we are also beginning to understand the social and environmental impact of our local action on distant ecosystems and economies. We prize hardwood for its natural beauty, but must now weigh its use against the extinction of species in distant rain forests. By the late 1980s, resource conservation efforts focusing on issues of social and environmental justice were competing for attention as the future of environmentally- and health-oriented action and practice.

The world is indeed bound fast by invisible cords. The way that we choose to see this tumultuous history is that each new crisis and each new response has opened our eyes to a larger world of interconnections. You can find books that were written at the turn of the last century that are similar to *Healthy by Design*. These also argue for proper siting and room layouts that recognize the position of the sun, and emphasize the need for good ventilation and adequately designed plumbing. Timeless design issues don't change but, at least in the industrialized world, the health and sanitation problems of the past have long since been resolved and enshrined in common practice and building codes. The horizons of good design have been further broadened by environmental concern. In the end good design involves a way of thinking that anticipates future problems as well as being mindful of current ones. This book takes the personal health of the occupant as its focus, but it does so with the idea of building on advances being made across all of the frontiers of environmentally responsible design.

—JAMES WASLEY, SEPTEMBER 1997

CHAPTER 1

Why a Healthy Home?

WHAT IS A HEALTHY HOME?

For most of us, ideal indoor conditions are similar to outdoor conditions during pleasant weather. A perfect home environment might feel like an orchard on a mild spring day, with gentle breezes blowing, limitless fresh air and subtle fragrances—there may be pleasant diffuse light passing through tree canopies, the sounds of rustling leaves, other people, and perhaps flowing water. This idyllic image suggests that the best building is like no building at all. But of course we need supportive shelter when the weather is harsh. However, instead of supportive shelter, many of us live and work in buildings filled with desiccated and stagnant air, surrounded by chemical vapors and hazardous dust, under monotonous lights, assaulted by a chaotic symphony of buzzing, clanking, growling, and squeaking equipment. These conditions are largely the result of poorly conceived, financially expedient building design. There is growing evidence that today's artificial environments are a major cause of irritation, stress and ultimately disease.

When we put up walls and a roof we are shaping an environment which can be measured against the best conditions provided by nature. How does your home or office compare to the shade of a tree on a mild, breezy day? Probably not very well. The healthy home should provide the best possible setting for people, with light and air, thermal comfort and freedom from excess noise, as well as appropriate and interesting spaces, lighting, color and textures. But the healthy home is not just for people; it can also be better for the earth.

By the broadest definition, energy and resource efficiency are also aspects of a truly healthful and wholesome house. A healthy home is not just a place free of hazards and toxins; rather it is a place that provides positive, life-affirming conditions in which its occupants can live and thrive, and which rests lightly on the earth.

In some respects the "natural ideal" is a romantic and impractical notion. The idea that all good things exist in nature and that a natural philosophy is the path back to innocence is naive and utopian. We will not all go back to the fields and forests again, nor would we all want to, but bringing some elements of the fields and forests back to our dwellings and workplaces is a means of healing the separation between humans and nature.

WHO NEEDS A HEALTHY HOME?

Healthy buildings aren't just for sick people. In this age of health consciousness a great deal of attention has been focused on diet, exercise and personal habits such as smoking and alcohol and drug use, but there is another, less apparent realm that may be affecting your health: your home and work environments. Everyone is affected to some extent. Just as about one-quarter of all people are considered "allergic" to environmental conditions in the usual sense, that is, they suffer from hay fever, asthma or other disorders triggered by plant materials, molds or animal dander, there are also people who are sensitive to chemical exposure. It is hard to say how many are affected, but it is likely that about one in three of us is sensitive to something in the environment, and will experience symptoms, often without knowing the source. In fact, recent health statistics indicate that the proportion of the young adult and adult population experiencing conventional allergies rose by about 8% (from 19% to 27%) in the 12 years prior to 1992.

Our home environment is vital to our health, especially in hot and cold weather. Homemakers, the very young and the very old spend up to 90% of their time inside. People working outside the home still spend about 50% of their time at home, indoors. Yet while public attention and government regulation have focused on the need to control environmental pollution, little has been said about indoor conditions and prevention.

A healthy home may play a key role in preventing health problems. You probably know at least one person with serious allergies who has put a special air filter in the home, removed carpets, or taken other measures to relieve respiratory suffering indoors. Or, you probably are aware of people installing sophisticated water filters, changing their lamps to full spectrum types, changing their windows to get more daylight, and trying to avoid exposure to electromagnetic fields from electrical equipment and power lines. Most people are doing these things, not because of a health problem, but because they are researching and thinking ahead. When we look back in

Healthy buildings are for prevention.

time, we see that many serious hazards, such as lead, DDT and asbestos, could have been avoided if more prudent and critical attitudes had prevailed. Isn't it time to apply more care to the future?

WHY THE CONCERN?

Concerns over healthy housing are well founded. Our lives today are more complex, stressful and difficult than ever before. Physical and emotional trauma and anxiety are daily conditions for many. Not one of us is immune to family problems, financial worries, safety concerns, and fears about the future of society and the environment. Another layer of stress from toxic or allergenic environmental exposures and poor living and working conditions can overload the immune system, leading to environmental sensitivity which can, in the long term, have serious consequences for sufferers and everyone close to them. Even when such a breakdown does not occur, continued exposure to toxic substances at low levels from poor environmental conditions, may have a role in some of the problems many accept as part of the aging process. Increases in minor skin conditions, inflammation, joint problems and respiratory difficulties are examples of this.

Some well-known indoor hazards, such as lead, asbestos and carbon monoxide, are toxic, while others, such as pollen, fungi and animal dander, are allergenic. But there are thousands of toxic and allergenic substances, plus a wide range of irritants which are not as well understood—substances such as pesticides, solvents, vapors from plastics, and glass and mineral

The chemical revolution promised a better future for all.

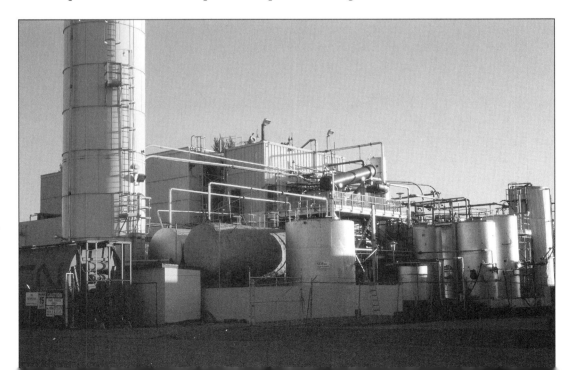

fibers. All of these are capable of causing chronic or acute illness, some in the short term, and others which may not appear for 20 years.

Examples of lesser known, harmful substances are formaldehyde, wood terpenes (vapors from softwood resins), paint solvents, and other gases and dusts which can mimic the effects of well-known allergens. They may cause similar symptoms to pollens and molds, such as congestion, shortness of breath, headaches, dizziness, loss of sleep and skin rashes. Prolonged exposure can lead to a decline in general health or specific disease. According to doctors who specialize in environmental illness, one effect caused by some substances is "sensitization." Exposure to formaldehyde or some types of wood dust, animal dander or molds, for instance, can incite immune reactions which will make people more sensitive to other gases, dusts or foods. Many people experience this immune sensitization as they age. This sensitizing process can, and often does, happen in the place which ought to be our sanctuary: our home.

Many recently identified syndromes, such as chronic fatigue, Epstein-Barr and candida seem to represent whole system failure. These syndromes affect a rapidly growing number of people, and are nearly always linked to immune system disorders, which strongly suggests that environmental factors are at work in these "new" diseases. It is probable that environmental stress is part of the entire picture of immune system overload which leads to a health breakdown, but environmental stressors are often missed or dismissed in diagnosis. A total health history, including environmental exposures at home and work can reveal conditions which are part of the problem, and which can be improved.

Chronic health conditions of this kind cause prolonged misery and anxiety, trips to various therapists, lost work time, family tension and stress. Some are treated with expensive medications when the source of the problem has not been identified. A problem which has been identified can be avoided. Removing or reducing the source from the environment should be part of total therapy and preventative action.

Those who are sensitized may find that, with reduction of sources, treatment and careful management, they can reach an equilibrium, and perhaps live a reasonably normal life. Some, if they act soon enough, can even avoid the total health collapse which many environmentally ill people experience, with its debilitating isolation, loss of physical and financial resources and abilities. In either case, sensitized people must be regarded as a special needs group, no different from those with impaired vision, hearing, mobility or mental capacity.

Poor environments have a role in stress and disease that is often overlooked by physicians.

4

THE VALUE OF COMFORT
AND PERSONAL CONTROL

We know intuitively that people must feel comfortable and in control of their immediate environment in order to be well, but we have done very poorly at delivering these conditions. Everyone has experienced a living or working situation in which the afternoon sun overheats one room terribly in the summer, where lighting is so poor that reading is difficult, where some rooms are never comfortable in winter, no matter what the thermostat setting, where noise from outside is inescapable, where the air is always stale or foul, or where there just isn't enough privacy for quiet relaxation. If a building is to be a refuge, control of these many factors is essential.

Control doesn't just mean having the right technology. Control relegated to machines is no control for many people. An indoor environment programmed to respond to sensors with preset thresholds for modulating light, air, heat, security, and appliance operation may appeal to those few who are fascinated with technology, and it may be helpful to those who are physically impaired, but for most of us it is just another layer of separation between us and real control over our environment. A window latch or light switch is a direct connection to a desired adjustment. It has an immediate and observable effect that is uncomplicated and satisfying.

The so-called "smart home," which is wired for many possible automated operations, may allow the busy commuter to turn on the oven to cook the dinner by using a cellular phone while stuck in traffic on the freeway, but such automation really doesn't help bring tangible and direct control over our environment back into our lives.

Another more appropriate means of environmental control is to design the building to passively respond to climate. Windows that admit sun when it is wanted, but are shaded in warm weather, openings that catch summer breezes, and walls that absorb unwanted noise are all part of good design. If those elements are created well, the technology to maintain control is simplified and minimized.

As well as allowing us direct control over our environment, our homes must also be a comfortable refuge.

Comfort encompasses more than well-fitted furniture. It also includes varied lighting which allows the eyes to work and to rest, fresh air which allows the lungs to function, freedom from annoying noise, pleasant temperatures, gentle air movement and humidity. When any of these comfort thresholds is exceeded, irritation results. At the other extreme, precise con-

Comfort requires control over your environment, but also variety.

trol is monotonous. Just as we expect the seasons to change, most of us need to feel differences in lighting and color, air movement and temperature. And these should be related to some natural phenomena, such as the weather or our movement through the building. A carefully designed and constructed home has features which prevent extremes of glare, temperature and air movement, excess noise and other irritants, while providing stimulation and interest. For example, a comfortable home might have a quiet, enclosed space with warm, subtle lighting, free from drafts with a warmer temperature, followed by a bold open space, with dramatic high-lighting, coolness and free air movement. A design stressing comfort and health may go much further and provide protection from invisible and poorly understood stressors such as electromagnetic fields.

Good design recognizes that health is much more than the absence of disease. It is also a sense of well-being supported by life-affirming conditions of light, comfort, space, color, and usually access to natural elements such as plants, trees, earth, stone, wood and water.

EVERY BUILDING A HEALTHY BUILDING?

We have been led to accept the idea that the home is the main private area in our lives, and that we should not expect the same environmental quality at work, at school, or in a store, restaurant or health clinic. But healthy building practices can be applied to workplaces, schools and other buildings. Every office or industrial shop with a personalized space, good control over lighting, air quality and noise, and a degree of privacy can expect improved occupant satisfaction and potentially, improved productivity and reduced sick time. As for classrooms, where could it be more important to be safe and comfortable and feel in control than in a learning environment? All that is lacking is the will of these institutions to make changes.

Businesses and professional practices are finding it makes financial sense to show more care and concern for the customer or client by providing more comfortable and interesting waiting or seating areas, better lighting, and no-smoking policies, even where it is not required by law. A reception area with art, plants, generous and interesting light, fresh air and a pleasant furniture arrangement sends a message—you are a welcome and important visitor. It might include a unique floor covering, an aquarium or any number of other features which make people stop and notice, and feel "at home."

By implementing these same principles workplaces, schools and other buildings can also be healthy.

6

CHAPTER 2

The History of the Healthy Home

From the cave we have advanced to roofs of palm leaves, of bark and boughs, of linen woven and stretched, and of grass and straw, of boards and shingles, of stones and tiles. At last, we know not what it is to live in the open air, and our lives are domestic in more senses than we think. From the hearth the field is a great distance. It would be well, perhaps, if we were to spend more of our days and nights without any obstruction between us and the celestial bodies. Let us learn from the poet who did not speak so much from under a roof, or the saint who did not dwell there so long. Birds do not sing in caves, nor do doves cherish their innocence in birdhouses. —HENRY THOREAU, *WALDEN*, 1854

Light and air have been understood as fundamental to health for centuries. Before the industrial age, life on a farm or in a village entailed a good deal of time spent outdoors. This was fortunate, because indoors was likely to mean dark, damp, smoke-filled rooms with little comfort. By the early 19th century, however, many people had left farm life for the city, and a factory job. The environment of the early industrial city was extremely unhealthy. Poisonous fog, contaminated water, crowding and disease were rampant. Tenement living was difficult, and workplaces usually worse. Children worked at very hazardous jobs, and people had a short life span, with an even shorter period of resilience and good health. By the mid-19th century, reformers began to work for safe and healthful living conditions. They wrote pamphlets and influenced legislation, and a few visionary industrialists even attempted to build "ideal communities." The physical foundations of these ideal places were light and air, quiet, open spaces, clean water and gardens—all of the elements lacking in the tenements. By the late 19th century, standards for protecting health and safety began to appear as labor codes, and eventually became part of building codes. All of our workplace safety standards, and the occupant safety components of building codes and design standards from which we benefit today, began in this period. Codes initially dealt only with prevention of fire, building collapse, and other matters of protecting life, but eventually expanded to include environmental quality matters such as daylight, room size, adequate heating and moisture control.

The 19th-century reaction against hazardous living conditions is at the root of today's healthy buildings and communities movement. Though living conditions are now very different, at least in the wealthier industrialized world, and technology and legal rights have advanced dramatically, fundamental human needs are the same, and the precepts of healthy living remain the same. Designing and building healthy buildings remains an attempt to regain the best qualities offered by nature, many of which have been lost through urbanization and industrialization. These qualities are still light, air, space, quiet, and a connection to nature and comfort.

THE OLD HOME

The idea that prewar or even 19th-century houses are healthy houses is a popular misconception, probably based on the knowledge that technology and modern materials and building practices are part of the sick building syndrome. This is partly true, but old homes have their own set of problems. They tend to be damp, musty, gloomy and noisy, erratically heated, and often filled with stale odors, mildew, asbestos, lead pipes and paint, as well as failing heating, cooling and ventilating equipment. Basements are often damp and rotting, dust is thick in every crack and hidden space, and faulty chimneys, old wiring and leaky gas appliances may represent serious hazards.

To add to this litany of problems, old homes often have small, awkward rooms, narrow stairs, too many doors and corridors, and they are usually not well insulated or weather sealed. Old homes usually lack ventilation and vapor barriers for moisture control, which are very important in cold climates. The only real exceptions are some well-crafted, climate-adapted old homes, usually pre-1940s, but these are rare. They may offer sheltered porches, generous windows, grand stairs, fine interior plaster and woodwork and high ceilings. However, if the heating, insulation, plumbing and electrical systems have not been upgraded, these houses are usually candidates for a lot of expensive work, particularly in the kitchen and bathrooms. Many older homes also have exterior woodwork or failing brickwork, which requires continual maintenance, windows that leak or get frosty in winter, crumbling foundations, flooding basements, pipes that gurgle and leak, and rooms always smelling of old wood and dust.

Older homes are not usually healthy homes, though they may be good candidates for remodeling.

8

In spite of all these problems, old homes are not all bad. There are possible air quality benefits to be found in an old home, particularly if you are considering major renovations. For example, the leaky construction probably allowed random ventilation and heat loss through wall and ceiling cavities which, if poorly insulated, are probably very dry and sound, even in a damp climate. Also, older materials, such as hardwood and tile, are safer than many new ones, such as wall-to-wall carpet and vinyl. But these are unreliable benefits, especially when weighed against the risks and unknowns in an older home.

DEVELOPMENTS IN HEALTHY HOUSING

Unfortunately, the new home-building methods and materials which solved many of the comfort and maintenance problems of old houses have led to a new set of problems. The older home was forgiving because it was loose and leaky. Any problems, such as excess moisture, chimney gases, cooking odors and emissions from materials, were less likely to make it unhealthy because they were not contained. But in a climate requiring heating or air conditioning, a loose, leaky building is very difficult to keep comfortable without an extraordinary amount of energy. Since the 1970s, not only

This house represents a culmination of healthy building developments. Energy and resource efficiency combine beautifully with health and style.

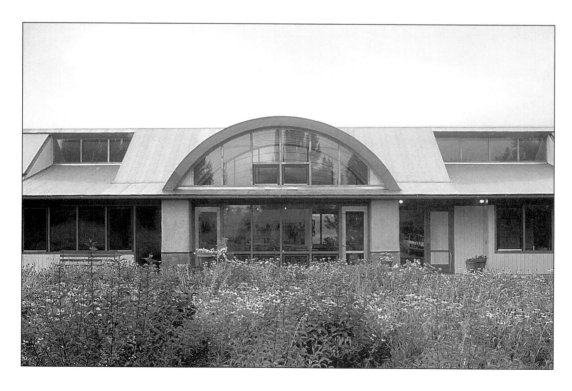

have our comfort expectations increased, but it has also become necessary to use energy more wisely and efficiently. We now have well-sealed houses which are more easily heated or cooled, but they are often dry and noisy, filled with chemical vapors, humming appliances, high maintenance floor coverings and harsh lighting.

Advances in technology have produced sick homes whose problems range from the mildly annoying to the very serious. An energy efficient home's fresh air supply through leakage is likely to be a small fraction of what it was in an old, drafty home. Therefore the exhaust and outdoor air needed to remove and dilute the products of combustion, cooking, respiration and the ever-present release of chemical vapors from household items, building materials, and finishes must be supplied by fans during heating or cooling periods. Unfortunately, adequate ventilation technology is still not mandated by most building codes, so it is not provided by builders. Even when provided, ventilation is not well understood or accepted by most homeowners or renters. And too often, ventilation is provided or added to attempt to make a building livable when it has serious air quality problems, particularly in cold winter conditions or during cooling season when it is tightly sealed. The only real freedom from this dilemma comes from locating homes in very mild regions where little heating or cooling is required throughout the year, and the windows can be left open.

Early efforts to adapt existing buildings and construction practices to comfort and energy-efficiency demands created some sick buildings, simply because the building was not understood as a whole system. Increasing insulation without increasing draft tightness can seriously damage insulated walls and ceilings in a heating or air-conditioning climate. And draft sealing without providing reliable, healthy ventilation can create a sick building. Consequently, building science had to adapt a whole system approach to building environments. The logical sequence of reasoning, based on the "systems principles" of building science for a cold climate or an air-conditioning climate results in this chain of decisions:

- To reduce energy use, increase comfort, and reduce interior moisture problems (such as condensation on cold window surfaces) in a cold climate, insulation levels in walls, ceilings and floors are increased beyond traditional, minimum amounts. The same is done in air-conditioning climates, though moisture generated indoors is usually not a problem.
- Higher insulation levels increase the likelihood of moisture problems inside insulated cavities, because lower temperatures can occur

there, and airborne moisture reaching the cavities will condense. This moisture can lead to rot, mold growth and reduced insulation performance, all of which are detrimental to indoor conditions and will damage interior or exterior finishes and structures. In an air-conditioning climate the damage is likely to occur near the inside surface. In a heating climate, it is likely to occur near the outside.

- With tighter draft sealing, the insulation value of the windows also needs to be improved to prevent condensation problems. With more insulation and better windows, though total energy use is lower, ventilation and air leakage now account for a larger portion of energy requirements, typically increasing from 30 percent for a conventionally insulated house in a cold climate, to over 50 percent for a well-insulated one.

- To protect insulated cavities from condensation, reduce heat losses by air leakage, and improve comfort, a continuous air barrier and a vapor barrier is incorporated in the insulated walls, floors, and ceilings. This has the added benefit of reducing the entry of outdoor air pollution (such as dust and pollen) and air pollutants such as dust and gases from materials inside the structural cavities. In a cold climate the vapor barrier is installed on the inside. In an air conditioning climate, it is done on the outside.

- Incorporating a continuous air barrier reduces air leakage, trapping moisture and pollutants in the building, potentially leading to poor indoor air quality and damage from high humidity levels. Though some indoor pollutants can be regulated at source, those which cannot, such as cooking odors, moisture from bathing, and body odors, will have to be extracted by an exhaust fan, and the remainder diluted by a reliable means of outdoor air ventilation. Due to the fact that natural ventilation is random, and driven largely by weather conditions, continuously operated, mechanical ventilation connected to all occupied rooms is considered the most reliable option for a cold climate or where air conditioning is necessary.

- The continuous operation of a mechanical ventilation system increases energy consumption, due to the requirement for heating and cooling of ventilation air, and the operation of fan motors.

In the 1970s mechanical design standards were changed to reduce the ventilation rate to save energy, particularly in commercial buildings, thus creating more sick buildings. To allow a higher ventilation rate, to help keep the building healthy without excessive energy use, a heat-recovery ventilator system is recommended for very cold or hot conditions. This device transfers the heat from indoor air as it leaves the building in winter to the incoming ventilation air. During air-conditioning periods, it transfers the heat from incoming outdoor air to the exhaust air, which is cooler.

The premises of building science and the emphasis on energy efficiency and comfort lead directly to the mechanically controlled house. This line of reasoning is now embedded in codes and practice in cold and hot climates. There is little doubt that the result can be comfortable, durable, energy efficient buildings, if it is all done well, but is it the only way to make healthy buildings? Are the results reliable, forgiving, and cost effective?

The "naturally conditioned house" is another alternative which is possible for most of the year in a very mild climate. The natural house approach is the opposite of the mechanically controlled house. It is as open to the breezes, sun and sky as it can be. It may have simple, movable shades for summer, loose-fitting windows, whole walls which open up, and little insulation or draft control. Heating may be a simple radiant unit with no ducts or filters, adequate for a few cold days, and it may have little or no mechanical ventilation. Of course, even a highly insulated and mechanically conditioned house in a severe climate can operate as a naturally conditioned house for the mild part of the year, if openings are placed carefully, and adequate insect screens and other essentials are provided.

Correctly applied, healthy building design and construction uses new technology, but in a very careful and selective way, responding to site, climate and other natural issues, and using materials and equipment which are appropriate to human needs and broader environmental goals. As in the 19th century, the intent is to provide generous light and air, sun and shade, quiet and comfort, through the placement and design of the building. If this is done correctly, dependence on mechanical support is reduced, and the relationship to climate, the landscape and the earth are emphasized.

We cannot go back to the drafty home of the last century. They are simply too uncomfortable, labor intensive and expensive to keep. Few modern homeowners want to live with the lack of comfort, high operating costs and maintenance of a genuine traditional home, especially in a very hot or cold climate. Expectations of a home are higher today, and people have less time to spare. Fortunately, new technology can be selectively combined with good design to produce houses that are healthy, comfortable and efficient.

Some sick buildings are created by poorly considered energy efficiency improvements.

12

CHAPTER 3

The Unhealthy Home

An unhealthy home can actually make occupants ill, even those who have no history of allergies, chemical sensitivities or weak immunity. Some of the most common risks are from unvented combustion gases, soil gases, severe fungus contamination from moisture problems, dust from outdoor and indoor sources or inadequate filtration, and organic vapors from new materials or maintenance practices. Other health risks include lead from old plumbing and paint, asbestos from pipe insulation, and glass or mineral fiber from leaking insulation cavities. And these are only the building-related hazards. Occupants, their activities, cleaning and maintenance practices, furniture and hobbies introduce yet another set of indoor pollution sources which may be more significant than the building-related sources.

According to the conventional medical model, there are two general categories of indoor environmental problems which negatively affect physical health: toxic or pathogenic conditions, and allergenic conditions.

Toxic or pathogenic conditions result from well-known health hazards such as lead, asbestos, carbon monoxide, bacteria, and viruses. Other less-well-known causes of pathogenic conditions include substances such as solvents and pesticides. All of these hazards can contribute to chronic or acute illness, such as skin, lung, liver or kidney disease, and even cancers, most of which do not appear for several years after exposure.

Allergenic conditions result from less potent hazards such as pollens, animal dander, dusts and fungus. All of these hazards are capable of producing immune responses, but people's susceptibility to allergens varies widely. Among affected individuals, allergies can cause misery and lead to a decline in health or the development of a distinct disease.

There are numerous links between these categories. Some hazards such as formaldehyde, a gas from glued wood products and fabrics, is both toxic and allergenic. Formaldehyde is a well-known irritant, causing immune-

13

like reactions in approximately 20% of people, even at very low levels. At higher levels it is very irritating to anyone. Formaldehyde has recently been identified as a potential cause of cancer. Ultimately the conventional medical distinction between pathogens and allergens may not be very useful. For example, there are numerous substances which are irritants but not specifically toxic and there is a wide range of sensitivity in the population. Dusts from concrete and gypsum board, and many gases emitted by carpets and other materials are typical irritants, but to some they may cause debilitating symptoms. Furthermore, recognized allergens, such as molds, may actually have much more serious effects than was previously thought. For example, chronic exposure to high levels of mold particles and odors may actually cause respiratory disease in previously healthy people. A broader medical view acknowledges that disease can be caused by multiple factors. Each factor is a stressor, and when the individual capacity to handle stress is exceeded, one or more systems will fail.

The list of potential irritants and toxins is growing rapidly with the proliferation of new synthetic chemicals in almost everything that surrounds us. This includes our clothing, bathing and drinking water, and the air we breathe. An alarming number of these agents are absorbed by the body, and some accumulate for long periods causing toxic or immune-like reactions. Others mimic chemicals which regulate body functions, causing "error responses." Testing requirements for new chemicals may be rigorous, but it is impossible to anticipate all of their potential long-term effects, some of which will not be discovered until years after their introduction and acceptance. The financial gain from successful new products makes them very attractive to develop, and creates political pressure to approve them for sale. It is sobering to think that chlorofluorocarbons, DDT and PCBs were all considered "miracle chemicals" when they were introduced. New markets and uses for them doubled every few months until they had a momentum that was hard to stop. As well as the chemicals used in agriculture and industry, building materials, furnishings and consumer products used in the home are important to our health and the environment. Developing and using them requires a great deal more care and scrutiny than has been exercised in recent decades if we are to avoid future problems. But materials are by no means the only factor in unhealthy buildings.

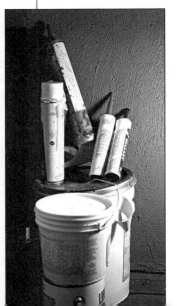

There are thousands of products now used in today's tightly sealed buildings which did not exist a few decades ago.

PROCESSES AND POLLUTANTS

There are a variety of processes and pollutants which can make buildings hazardous environments. Some enter from outside and some come from inside. The following are the major chemical and physical processes which produce contaminants inside the home.

Moisture

Breathing, cooking and washing all release moisture into the building where it remains until it is removed and replaced by outdoor air or cooling. Exhaust ventilation near the source of moisture is the best means of control when outdoor air is dryer than indoor. When outdoor air is saturated, as it often is in summer in a humid region, ventilation does not dry the building. Under these conditions, an air conditioner or dehumidifier may be used to dry indoor air. Plenty of air movement will also help where appropriate. Excess humidity indoors allows fungi and bacteria to reproduce, and airborne bacteria and viruses to survive longer, and possibly transmit disease.

At the other extreme, very dry conditions are irritating to the bronchia and skin, and cause dust to be easily released and suspended in the air. Bronchial drying causes respiratory difficulty in sensitive people, and is also thought to increase the risk of catching colds and flus. The ideal relative humidity is between 30% and 60%. Relative humidity is the measure of how much moisture air contains, compared to how much it could hold if fully (100%) saturated at that temperature. This can be easily measured with an inexpensive instrument (see Environmental Testing later in this chapter).

In very cold weather, or in desert regions in summer, the air may become excessively dry indoors, simply because there is little moisture outdoors. In these conditions, some form of humidification is often helpful. The simplest means in winter is to place pans of water on a warm surface. If an automatic humidifier is used and connected to a forced-air system, it is essential to keep it clean and free of leaks. It should be shut off when not needed, and cleaned before starting up. If it has a wick or wet fabric element, it should be replaced if it becomes discolored. Humidifiers are easily contaminated with fungus or hazardous bacteria. A wickless, ultrasonic or steam humidifier is safer. Humidification is generally not necessary unless the indoor level routinely falls below approximately 20%.

Combustion

Burning anything in the home consumes oxygen and produces vapors and air contaminants which range from minor irritants to asphyxiants and carcinogens. The most hazardous products are carbon monoxide and the aromatic compounds present in soot and tars, especially from wood and oil combustion.

It is essential that all fuel-burning furnaces, fireplaces and water heaters have a reliable combustion air supply, combustion chambers which are as well-sealed as possible, and reliable, fire-safe chimneys which will not leak into the building. The safest type of device is a "sealed combustion" unit. These have combustion air piped into a sealed chamber where the flames are. The exhaust gases are carried outdoors by a sealed pipe.

Warning: Unvented gas fireplaces, gas space heaters, propane construction heaters, catalytic heaters and kerosene heaters are potentially very unsafe and should not be used in tightly sealed or poorly ventilated buildings.

Outgassing / Offgassing

Evaporation which occurs in solids rather than liquids is called outgassing or offgassing. It is the slow release of chemicals which are components of the material, or of various treatments it has received. Some outgassing is a by-product of reactions going on within or at the surface of the material. These may be incomplete reactions among chemicals used in manufacturing or chemical residues, intentional or accidental. Paints, plastics and adhesives are usually the main sources of outgassing. Outgassing can be increased by moisture, heat, sunlight or the presence of other chemicals. It can be reduced by tightly enclosing the material in nonpermeable veneers, such as plastic or metal, or by sealing it with oil paints or vapor-resistant varnishes. This tends to capture the gases and slow their release. Outgassing decreases over time, but it may take some materials months or years to fully stabilize.

The products of outgassing are volatile organic compounds (VOCs). These are called volatile because they form vapors at room temperatures, and organic because they are chemical compounds based on carbon and hydrogen atoms, the same class of structures that are the basis of all life.

Some chemicals are classed as semi-volatile organic compounds (SVOCs). These are released more slowly than VOCs, and may outgas for years. Carpet backings, asphalt compounds, flexible vinyl flooring and upholstery covers, some paints, oils and varnishes, and plastic foams are materials which commonly contain semi-volatile compounds.

VOC's are generally irritants or neurotoxins. If they become concentrated in the air we breathe, they cause symptoms such as burning eyes, shortness of breath, headaches, dizziness and confusion. It is best to choose materials which have minimum offgassing potential, and to ventilate well while painting or using adhesives of the safest type available. (See Chapter 9, Materials).

Electromagnetic fields are poorly understood and controversial as a health issue.

16

Biological Activity

Microorganisms such as fungi (mildew and other molds) and bacteria can reproduce easily at room temperatures whenever moisture is present. All that molds need for nutrition is the slightest accumulation of dust, food, waste, a urine spill, damp wood, fabric or carpet. Fungi are very allergenic, and produce many gases which give them their characteristic odors. The gases are irritating to anyone, and possibly debilitating to sensitive people. The particles cause inflammation of the throat, nose and sinuses, and sometimes skin rashes in people with specific allergies. When dry, the fungi break up and release spores (seedlike particles) and other dust when they are disturbed. Walking over a moldy floor surface in dry conditions is a common way for particles to become airborne. It is important to remember that fungi are not just a risk to allergic people. Regular or massive exposure to fungal particles can cause previously healthy people to become allergic.

Bacteria produce odors and are primarily a nuisance. Fortunately, most dangerous bacteria are transmitted between people, not on interior surfaces in buildings. The main exceptions are the lethal bacteria, such as the type which causes Legionnaire's Disease, that can develop in very warm standing water, such as in the drain pans of humidifiers or air-conditioning systems. They can also develop in poorly maintained hot tubs and water heating systems. Of course, other well-known bacteria, such as those causing tuberculosis or pneumonia, are also easily transmitted through the air.

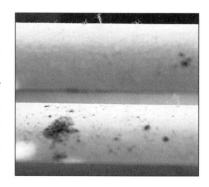

Preventing moist conditions, and cleaning the areas where dust and spills accumulate, is an effective prevention for fungus and surface bacteria. There are also some safe treatments, such as hydrogen peroxide followed by borax, which will clean up and retard future fungus growth.

Accumulated dust will support fungus growth when it becomes moist, even on metal window blinds.

Dust mites are another allergenic biological problem. These microscopic insects thrive wherever moisture is present, such as in bedding and upholstery. Mites and their droppings are a major cause of dust allergy, particularly in young children. Airing out bedding regularly, tumbling it in a hot dryer, and covering mattresses, cushions, pillows, and quilts with a special, tightly woven cloth called "barrier cloth" helps reduce exposure.

Adsorption

Adsorption is the physical attachment of a gas to a surface. It is not a chemical interaction, such as when baking soda absorbs odors in the refrigerator,

17

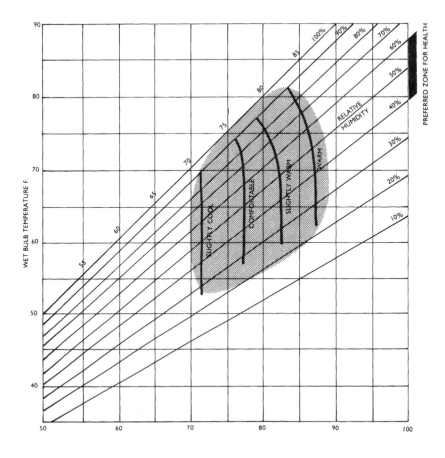

DRY BULB TEMPERATURE

Relative Humidity and Comfort

Comfort is dependent on both temperature and relative humidity. The shaded zone indicates the usual range of comfortable temperature and humidity for light activity when the air movement is moderate. Read room temperature on the bottom scale and humidity on the diagonal scale. Note that the preferred humidity zone for health is between 40% and 60%. (Adapted from *American Society of Heating, Refrigeration, and Air Engineers Fundamentals Handbook*.)

Note: To determine relative humidity from temperature measurements, locate dry bulb temperature on the bottom scale and wet bulb temperature on the left hand scale. Trace the vertical and horizontal lines to their meeting point and read the humidity from the diagonal scale. A wet bulb thermometer has a moistened sleeve placed over the end to cool it by evaporation.

Some recognized allergens, such as molds, may actually have much more serious effects than was previously thought.

18

and it is reversible. Many indoor surfaces trap air contaminants by adsorption and then release them slowly. Moisture, nitrogen oxides from combustion, and most organic vapors (VOCs) from offgassing, as well as odors from cooking, smoking and hobbies are adsorbed and then released this way. This effect explains why buildings smell of smoke or cooked food long after the source is gone and the air changed. Carpet, drapery, upholstery and plaster have a high adsorption ability. Vinyl, ceramic, finished wood, glass and metals have little ability to adsorb. Due to the adsorption effect, it is very important to ventilate well whenever paint, adhesive or volatile cleaners are used to reduce the high concentration of volatiles which aid adsorption onto surfaces. It is also important to "flush out" buildings after construction, and before occupancy, by excess ventilation.

Material Deterioration

All common materials break down over time. Textiles such as carpets, upholstery, bedding and draperies eventually begin to lose their fiber structure and shed small particles. Paints and varnishes begin to lose their color and become brittle. Soft plastics shrink, become hard and eventually crack. These processes are accelerated by sunlight and high temperatures, and sometimes by moisture. In many cases, fibers and gases are released into the air as the materials deteriorate. Metals, ceramics, glass and porcelain are very stable and do not deteriorate. Wood deteriorates very slowly.

Protecting vulnerable materials from sunlight and heat will extend their lives and reduce the release of fibers and gases. The safest materials for use where sunlight, heat and moisture are expected are the very inert ones: metals, glass and ceramics.

Electromagnetic Fields

Electromagnetic fields are a special class of potential hazards. They have only recently been recognized as risks, and are now being more fully studied. Of all the indoor pollution sources listed, electromagnetic fields are the most controversial.

All electrical equipment is surrounded by electrical and magnetic fields of varying strengths and types, and the chemical activity inside the living cell, and the nerve and fluid exchanges in the body all operate by electrochemical activity. Because the fields from electrical equipment can induce electrical changes in body tissues, it has been known for some time that strong fields influence health. Until the mid-1970s, however, the low-frequency, low-strength electrical fields from power lines, appliances and other common technology around buildings were not considered health

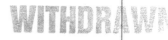

risks. Only exposure to high-frequency, highpowered equipment, such as radar and broadcasting stations, was linked to disease, and only among those working close to it. The belief was that only a field strong enough to cause heating in tissues could cause damage.

Since that time, laboratory research and studies of human populations have convinced many that even low-level electromagnetic fields produced by electrical services to buildings and common devices such as televisions, computers, electric blankets and electric appliances may have a health risk. The likely effects of exposure are greater fatigue and mental stress, a loss of immune function causing greater susceptibility to illness, and possibly increased risk of cancers, particularly leukemia and certain nerve and brain tumors. Though the evidence is not conclusive, the International Agency for Research on Cancer (IARC) Special Working Group on Non-Ionizing Radiation has concluded that there is a probable correlation between risk of many cancer types and lowfrequency field exposure. It stops short of suggesting a mechanism for how this occurs, but supports the conclusion that "prudent avoidance" is a wise precaution for everyone.

Life on earth evolved with only the earth's magnetic field and minor static electrical activity as electrical influences. Today we are surrounded by high-voltage lines, transformers and substations, transmitters, building wiring, appliances and many other sources of these fields. The problem is to determine what types of fields should be of concern, and what can be done about them.

Electrical and Magnetic (Inductive) Fields

There are two field types: electrical fields and magnetic (inductive) fields. An electrical field can be illustrated as the difference in charge between a cloud and the earth which may result in lightning. It is measured in volts per foot or volts per meter. These fields are present in our bodies when walking across a carpet on a dry day, by being near high-voltage wiring, or by being near or touching objects such as televisions which carry a charge. Many of these fields are direct current (DC) and are relatively constant, and therefore are not thought to be as active in living tissues as the magnetic fields from alternating current (AC) sources which change direction or oscillate rapidly. Electrical fields are very easy to shield. Isolating the source with an insulator, or placing a conductive shield over the source and connecting it with a wire to a grounding system will effectively control electrical fields. A grounded shield placed over a computer monitor is an example of electrical shielding. However, it does not shield the magnetic component.

Prudent avoidance is the best strategy for electro-magnetic fields in the absence of conclusive health evidence.

Magnetic fields are generated by any current flow in an electrical conductor. The magnetic field around an electric motor or wire, or the magnetic energy radiating from a cordless or cellular phone, a television or computer monitor, or broadcasting station, or a microwave oven are all examples. These fields are different from electrical fields because they will induce electrical currents in objects within their range, including living organisms, without having to touch them. Magnetic fields are AC, meaning they reverse positive and negative polarity many times each second, and therefore induce alternating currents in objects nearby. Magnetic fields are measured in units of Gauss, or tesla. These magnetic fields cannot be shielded by normal means, the way electrical fields can, because they are capable of radiating magnetic energy through even steel or concrete. Distance is one reliable method of reducing exposure; the only other practical means is to redesign the electrical device to cancel some of the fields. This has been done with electric blankets and radiant heating panels recently. The two conductors carrying current have been located closer together so that their opposite fields tend to cancel each other. Computer monitors have also been redesigned to reduce their magnetic fields.

There are many complex characteristics to magnetic fields which probably determine their biological effects, such as strength, frequency, pulse rate (if they are pulsed) and polarity in relation to the earth's magnetic field. Most attention is currently focused on fields classed as Extremely Low Frequency (ELF), which is between 0 and 100 hertz (cycles per second), because these are the fields common around most devices operated by household electricity. Higher frequency fields also occur around computers, televisions, microwave ovens, cordless and cellular phones, and other equipment.

Their complex characteristics make them more difficult to study. There are at least four ways electrical and magnetic fields act on living things which may explain their effects on health and well-being. These have all been observed in laboratory experiments or human population studies:

- Effects on chemical exchanges in cells, such as calcium absorption
- Effects on chemicals which regulate nerve and brain activity, such as serotonin and melatonin, which are important in stress release and sleep
- Suppression effects on immune cells, leading to increased illness and possibly cancer
- Direct changes to DNA and DNA repair mechanisms, possibly leading to mutation and cancer

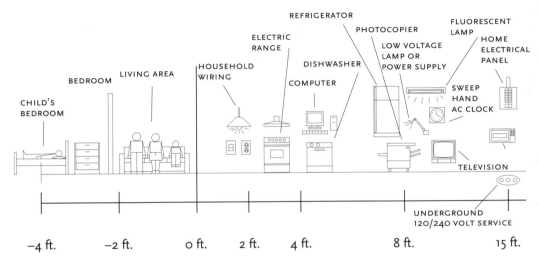

Magnetic Field Exposure Avoidance

All power lines and appliances produce magnetic fields which are suspected contributors to stress and disease. Correcting certain wiring faults can reduce the fields, but distance is the only reliable avoidance method. These fields cannot be practically shielded. The suggested distances are based on maintaining exposure below 1.5 mG (milligauss) from that source, based on fields from a stronger than average device. Note that bedrooms and children's areas should be further removed than less occupied areas.

Some scientists active in electrical health research simply summarize that these fields place stress on living organisms, and can therefore have direct and indirect consequences on health and well-being. It is likely that high-frequency fields, such as those from radio transmitters, are more strongly linked to the most serious health risks than low-frequency fields from power lines and building wiring.

Environmental health exposure standards are all based on guesswork, and electromagnetic field exposure standards are the most difficult to verify, so most countries have been reluctant to adopt them. In Sweden and Russia there are recommended maximum exposure standards for magnetic fields,

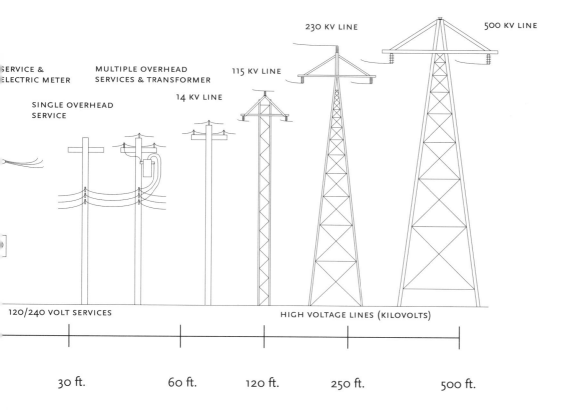

SERVICE &
ELECTRIC METER

SINGLE OVERHEAD
SERVICE

MULTIPLE OVERHEAD
SERVICES & TRANSFORMER

14 KV LINE

115 KV LINE

230 KV LINE

500 KV LINE

120/240 VOLT SERVICES

HIGH VOLTAGE LINES (KILOVOLTS)

30 ft.   60 ft.   120 ft.   250 ft.   500 ft.

based on the limits suggested by research. In many other places, health authorities are now discussing possible actions with city planning departments and electrical utility companies. Some courts in the United States have recognized the risk and have ordered electrical equipment moved, and even awarded damages to claimants in a few situations.

Sweden has also recently instituted a maximum magnetic field emission standard for computer monitors, based on extensive studies of office workers in data centers who use them daily. This standard is now accepted around the world, and is indicated by a "Low Radiation" seal on the monitor. It is not a guarantee of safety, but simply a prudent precaution to lower potential risk to the user and people nearby.

For building wiring, household and office equipment, electrical service lines to buildings, transformers, substations and high-voltage lines, distance is the only reliable protection from magnetic fields. The figure above indicates the approximate distance required to maintain exposure below the Swedish computer monitor standard using an "above average to worst case" field from each common source. Please note that children's and adults' bedrooms should be further away than other living and working spaces to further reduce exposure.

23

TABLE OF COMMON AIR POLLUTANTS

NAME	SOURCES	EFFECTS	CONTROL
excess moisture	cooking, washing, breathing	increases fungus, bacteria and dust mite growth	exhaust ventilation, dehumidification, air conditioning. Too little moisture also affects health.
carbon dioxide	human respiration	minor discomfort at high levels, feelings of "stuffiness"	CO_2 level is a good indicator of ventilation rate in tightly enclosed spaces (e.g. bedrooms), or where occupancy is high (e.g. schools, offices)
carbon monoxide	incomplete combustion in furnaces, stoves and fireplaces	headaches, dizziness, sleepiness, muscle weakness, potentially lethal	safe chimneys, sealed combustion burners
nitrogen oxides	high temperature combustion	irritation, possible immune suppression	safe chimneys, sealed combustion burners
sulfur oxides	burning of fuels containing sulfur, e.g. oil, coal	potent irritant, burning eyes, reduces lung function	alternative fuels, safe chimneys, sealed burners
polynuclear aromatic hydrocarbons	smoking, combustion of wood and coal, barbecuing, burnt food	irritants and carcinogens	prohibit smoking, use clean fuels, burn dry wood only in enclosed firebox and don't restrict oxygen, use low temperature cooking
ozone	laser printers, photocopiers, small "brush type" motors, electronic air cleaners	inflammation of bronchia, wheezing and shortness of breath, dizziness, asthma attacks	remove or exhaust sources, maintain electronic air cleaners

NAME	SOURCES	EFFECTS	CONTROL
formaldehyde	particle board, interior laminated and decorative panels, glues, fabric treatments, paints, and many other items	burning eyes and nose, skin rash, shortness of breath, headaches, nausea, dizziness, fatigue	use alternative, safer materials, seal particle board which can't be removed, ventilate
volatile organic compounds (VOCs) other than formaldehyde	paints, solvents, carpets, soft plastics, adhesives, caulkings, softwoods, paper products, cleaning and maintenance products	intoxication, burning eyes or nose, shortness of breath, headaches, dizziness, nausea, loss of judgment, panic	use alternative, safer materials, age materials before installing, ventilate
lead	old paint (pre-1970s), pipes and solder (pre-1985), dust and soil from beside roads (residue from leaded gas)	neurotoxic, especially if ingested by young children. Learning disabilities, nausea, trembling, numbness of fingers and toes.	identify and remove or seal old paint (expert advice may be necessary), replace pipes and solder with lead-free, avoid foods grown by roadside
pesticide residues	treated basements and foundations, treated wall and ceiling cavities, treated cabinets and closets, treated soil outside foundation. *Note:* pre-1980s treatments are more likely to leave residues and be toxic.	neurotoxic or long-term risk of liver, kidney and other disease, including cancers	identification and removal by qualified expert if history known, sealing pesticide in if possible

25

TABLE OF COMMON AIR POLLUTANTS (continued)

NAME	SOURCES	EFFECTS	CONTROL
asbestos fiber	steam pipe and duct insulation (pre-1975), furnace and fireplace parts, reinforced vinyl floor tile (pre-1980), fiber cement shingles and siding (pre-1980)	long-term cancer risk from breathing fibers	do not disturb material, get expert identification and removal if required, seal with special sealant and cover with sheet metal if not crumbling
mineral and glass fiber	thermal insulation, pipe insulation, fire-resistant acoustic tile and fabrics	potent irritant, burning eyes, itching skin, long-term risk of lung damage and cancer	handle only with respirator and gloves, seal and enclose. Do not disturb in place.
fungus particles, dust mites	grow in basements, damp carpet, bedding, fabrics, walls and ceilings, closets	very allergenic, burning eyes and nose, sneezing, skin rash, congestion and shortness of breath	keep surfaces dry and clean, cover bedding and upholstery with barrier cloth, ventilate, use borax treatments to retard fungus
hazardous bacteria (e.g. legionella)	standing warm water, untreated hot tubs, air-conditioning drain pans, humidifier reservoirs	cause severe respiratory illness, potentially lethal	prevent standing water, clean and treat tubs and humidifier reservoirs.
radon gas, methane and other soil gases	radon: natural radioactivity in soils. Others: decomposing garbage in landfills or toxic waste	radon: increased lifetime lung cancer risk. Others: possibly toxic or explosive, nuisance odors	know site history before building, remove soil if necessary, seal foundation and floor drains, ventilate subsoil if necessary

ENVIRONMENTAL TESTING

Testing for and measuring air pollution indoors can be quite complicated and expensive. The only relatively simple tests are for humidity, carbon monoxide, carbon dioxide, formaldehyde, radon and fungal spores. Testing for other volatile organic compounds, pesticides, hazardous fibers and dusts, and so on, is very complex and must be done by a qualified specialist using sophisticated laboratory equipment.

Humidity can be measured with a hygro-thermometer (about $20 US), available at hardware and electronics stores. 30% to 60% is the ideal range for indoor humidity.

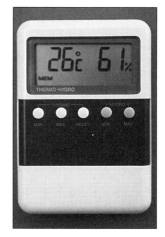

Carbon monoxide can be detected when it reaches unsafe levels by an alarm costing $35 to $100 US, similar to a smoke detector. These are available at building supply and hardware stores. One of these should be installed where there is a fuel-burning device with a conventional chimney, particularly if the building is thoroughly draft sealed and has any large exhaust fans. Not all are effective, however; it is wise to check consumer testing results before buying.

Carbon dioxide can be measured as an indicator of ventilation rate in enclosed spaces. This is really only useful in occupied classrooms, meeting rooms and office areas. Most homes have few occupants, so CO_2 measurements are usually not very useful. Measurement requires an "infrared spectrometer" available only from specialized instrument suppliers. The cost is about $700 to $1200 US for a device for CO_2 only. The outdoor level is 350 ppm (parts per million). Below 800 ppm indoors indicates reasonably good ventilation. Above 1200 ppm indicates poor ventilation.

An inexpensive hygro-thermometer will monitor indoor humidity and help to assess ventilation, dehumidification or humidification needs.

Formaldehyde can be measured with a sampler which is exposed to the air and then returned to the manufacturer for analysis. Most air pollution laboratories in major cities can provide these. The cost is about $35 US per test. Levels below 0.05 ppm are very safe. Between 0.05 ppm and 0.10 ppm indicates potential irritation. Any level above 0.15 ppm suggests action should be taken to identify and reduce sources.

Radon can be measured with a sampler available from specialized suppliers or air pollution measurement laboratories. The electret or film types are best, and cost about $35 US each. Sampling with activated carbon is not reliable. Two samplers should be exposed for several months, especially over a winter season, one in the basement, and one in a bedroom or living room. In the United States, the action level (the level at which some steps should be taken to reduce exposure) set by the Environmental Protection Agency is above 4 pCi/L (picocuries per liter). Because radon is a long-term risk, action is not urgent unless the level is extremely high. The action level in Sweden and Canada is much higher at 20 pCi/L.

Fungal spores can be sampled using sterile plates containing a nutrient mixture, available from specialized suppliers or air pollution laboratories at a modest cost. These are exposed for about one hour in rooms at breathing level, then covered and incubated for several days. The spores which bloom on the plate can be observed to give a rough indication of fungal dust levels. Identification of the type of fungus is recommended where extreme sensitivity or severe contamination is suspected, but this can only be done by an expert mycologist. This method does not allow an accurate count of the number of spores. To do so requires an air pump type sampler.

Water testing should be done before deciding what, if any, treatment is necessary, unless it is municipal water and its contents are well known. A basic water test costs about $25 US. It can cost much more, depending on what tests are requested. A water quality expert or public health officer should be consulted for specialized advice.

Electromagnetic fields can be measured with a simple field strength meter, available from specialty suppliers for about $50 to $250 US, depending on features. One can also be rented by the day or week from some makers and specialty services. Generally, magnetic fields should be below about 2 mG (milligauss) for sleeping and living areas, though this has not been well established. See the Electromagnetic Fields section earlier in this chapter for more detail.

Light and lighting is primarily a design and quality matter. Measurement of light levels is not very useful, except for workplaces and public areas where regulations might specify a minimum illumination level for safety.

Noise measurement is also fairly simple, requiring a sound level meter available for purchase or rental from electronics stores and specialty suppliers.

A basic meter is about $150 US. Better ones may cost several hundred dollars. Sound is measured on a decibel (dB) scale using frequency bands and weightings. The most common scale for general noise measurement is dBA (decibels, A scale). Noise may be measured to compare conditions with industrial safety standards (to guard against hearing loss), residential comfort standards used in some municipal ordinances, or to make a legal case regarding nuisance noise.

Air Leakage Testing

One last, simple test procedure for buildings is testing to determine the amount of air leakage and where it is located. A new or existing building in a heating or air-conditioning climate which will have high insulation levels must be free from large leakage paths which allow moist air into insulated spaces. The best way to measure this is with a "fan door test." The fan door is a replacement door, installed in place of an outside door, which contains a powerful fan.

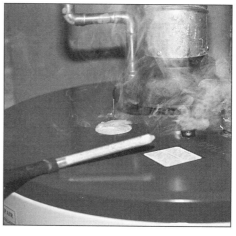

The door is installed temporarily, then intentional openings such as fireplace flues, exhaust fan ducts and clothes dryer vents are plugged. When the fan is started, it forces air into the building until the indoor air pressure rises to a set level. The relationship between fan speed and pressure indicates how much leakage area the building has. This is called "equivalent leakage area" (ELA), and is expressed as square inches or square centimeters of total cracks and leaks in the building. The leakage area can be divided by the total surface area of the building's outside walls and ceilings to arrive at a "normalized leakage area" (NLA), expressed as leakage area (square inches or centimeters) per unit of wall and ceiling area (square feet or meters). Normalized leakage area is a good indicator of the draft tightness of construction, and is often used in healthy and energy efficient building programs to determine construction quality.

Once the leakage area is measured this way, the fan can be reversed, causing the building to leak outdoor air through cracks. These cracks can then be located using a "smoke tube" device which makes artificial smoke. It is usually used along the baseboards, around windows and doors, and near electrical outlets, and plumbing and wiring in insulated walls, to determine where draft sealing improvements are needed.

A smoke tube indicates leakage of combustion gases from this water heater when the kitchen exhaust is operated with the home tightly sealed.

29

When to Test

Air quality testing is usually not necessary for a building if it has been designed and built with healthy building principles. If it has been built for a hypersensitive person, that person is a far more sensitive judge of conditions than most testing instruments. A sick building, or existing building which is to be remodeled, is often tested before improvements are begun to determine how successful changes are in improving air quality.

The other reason for testing is where a hazard such as radon or asbestos may exist which has no apparent effects in the short term. Radon testing is the only reliable way to determine if radon reduction repairs are needed in an existing building, because radon exposure has no symptoms, and radon cannot be detected by the senses.

Asbestos and lead are examples of risks which will affect the remodeling of older buildings, and which can only be determined by laboratory tests. If pipe insulation contains asbestos, or paint contains lead, handling or removing it is very risky and should be done only under very controlled conditions, by a qualified expert.

THREE STEPS TO REDUCTION

There are three basic steps which can be taken to reduce indoor pollution.

- First, eliminate the source whenever possible. When you have a choice, make careful selections of building materials, furnishings, paints, carpets and fabrics. Ceramics, metals, glass, concrete, plaster, hardwoods, and natural fiber cotton and wool are generally the safest materials. "Zero VOCs" rated interior paints are generally safe to handle, though special hypoallergenic paints may be necessary for the very sensitive. Alkyd "oil" paints are generally acceptable for outdoor use, and for specialized indoor use once they have cured, but a low-odor thinner should be used for cleanup, and it should be reused as much as possible. But be cautious, because alkyd paints may take several months or longer to reach an acceptable odor level. Use electricity for cooking where possible, and avoid indoor combustion which is not in a fully enclosed fire chamber. Reduce the use of cleaning, personal care and hobby products containing chlorine, solvents, perfumes and other volatile materials. Buy furniture wisely, avoiding particle boards and soft plastics, and minimize upholstery, draperies and carpets in areas where dust sensitivity is a problem.

- Second, seal or encapsulate any source of pollution you cannot remove, such as the particle board in newer kitchen cabinets or furniture, or exposed mineral, glass fiber or cellulose insulation. Small amounts of asbestos tape on the outside of ducts can be covered with a heat-resistant foil tape to prevent it from decaying and shedding. If the building has an air filtration system, install the best performance filters that can be used with that system. (See Air Filters in chapter 8.)

- Third, dilute any remaining air quality problems by improved ventilation. Improved ventilation is effective for reducing the concentration of nearly all harmful gases, except for those which may be more concentrated outdoors, due to air pollution in urban areas, or near industry or agriculture. Every kitchen, bath and laundry should have quiet, reliable exhaust fans, and they should be used regularly to remove smoke, odors and excess moisture. In a modern, draft-sealed home, every occupied room should have supply ventilation ducted to it and operable windows for mild weather.

- And finally, pay attention to those who have sensitivities. They have something to tell us all about prevention. Some sensitive people were not born that way, but became ill through exposure.

CHAPTER 4

The Spectrum of Concern

If it is asserted that civilization is a real advance in the condition of man, and I think that it is, though only the wise improve their advantages, it must be shown that it has produced better dwellings without making them more costly; and the cost of a thing is the amount of what I will call life which is required to be exchanged for it, immediately or in the long run.

—HENRY THOREAU, *ON WALDEN POND*

THE STAR DIAGRAM

The star diagram shown below illustrates the three main concerns when designing the healthy house: health, resource efficiency and energy efficiency.

Health is the personal part of healthy buildings. The question of what conditions are best for human health is the focus of this book. Resource efficiency is a more regional and global concern. What materials will this building require? What will they take from the earth? Are the materials renewable, plentiful and recycled? How much water and land will the building use? Energy efficiency is a global and regional concern. How small can the energy impact of this building be? How self-sufficient can it be, and how much will it cost to operate in the future? Each of the case studies that follow in this book is accompanied by a star diagram which shows its primary emphasis.

STANDARD PRACTICE

The Health Emphasis

To some degree, it is possible to make health an emphasis in all building design. Healthy buildings by design are not just for "special needs groups."

They are a wise investment in quality, comfort, and prevention for all.

Health may become a major priority on a project for several reasons. One or more of the occupants may have special health needs, such as extreme allergies or hypersensitivity. People with compromised immunity due to illness such as HIV, or as a result of cancer therapy or organ transplant, also need a carefully controlled environment. Often, air quality will be the major emphasis in these cases.

Another situation in which health may be a major priority is when the occupants are a group for whom prevention is paramount, as in classrooms for young children. Children are more likely to be allergic than adults because their body immunity has not stabilized, which it tends to do later in life. The young child's experience in the classroom is very important to future education success. The quality of the classroom environment in terms of light, color, space, air and sound is strongly emphasized by many educators for this reason.

Another special group may be people with emotional disorders or handicaps which make them extremely sensitive to light, noise and indoor air

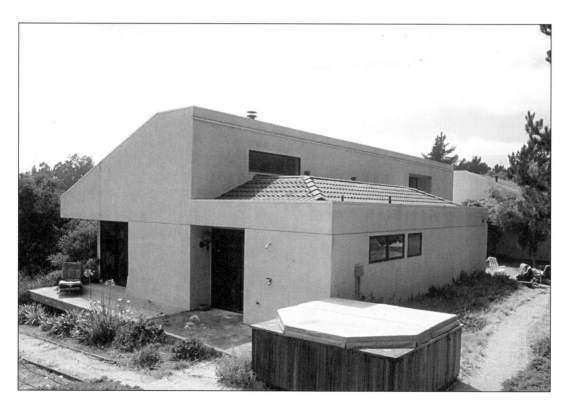

A gracious home that is also a healthy home on the northern California coast.

33

pollution. In the case of a group home, or day-use facility for a special needs group, careful control of the indoor environment may increase the success of the program.

Finally, the space may be used by the public, including those with special needs or communicable diseases. Medical clinics or social services offices are good examples of this. Paying close attention to environmental quality in these situations will help to make visitors and staff more comfortable, protect them from disease transmission, and send the message that the client and services are important.

In the star diagram used in the case studies in this book, the length of the health axis indicates how much healthy building design was emphasized in the project, according to the author's assessment and the information provided by the design team or owners. If there is no health emphasis shown on the diagram, the project is typical of conventional design, where health is only considered as far as is necessary to meet basic code requirements. If the diagram shows a full health emphasis, the project can be considered highly advanced or "state of the art."

The Energy Conservation Emphasis

Energy is a fundamental environmental currency. Those who have it are wealthy; those who don't are poor. Energy divides the world into haves and have-nots and is increasingly a cause for conflict and war. Energy-rich societies pour vast amounts of oil and electricity into automobiles, airplanes, buildings and consumer products; energy-poor societies use animal power and burn wood and agricultural waste to survive. In the late 20th century, it is finally becoming clear that even the wealthy cannot afford to be wasteful, and that wastefulness is not a necessary by-product of wealth. Not only is consumption a questionable path to a high quality of life, but wealthy societies are actually technologically best equipped to conserve.

In the building sector, the conservation ethic began to surface in the 1960s in the form of solar building designs and independent energy production. The momentum accelerated in the mid-1970s during the OPEC oil embargo, when we were all suddenly made aware of our dependency on oil. Since then, design knowledge has advanced to the point where a residential or commercial building can easily be designed to operate with less than half of the energy its equivalent would have used only 15 years ago, while providing a similar, or better, indoor climate.

Energy conservation in building design usually starts with the site, building form and orientation, seeking to optimize sunlight, daylight and

An energy efficient building is usually a very comfortable and durable building, with reduced maintenance needs.

wind. Once the best access to, and shelter from, these natural energies has been determined, the building envelope is considered. The windows, insulation, foundation, wall and roof materials, and use of thermal storage are all matched to the climate and intended interior uses and conditions. Finally, the actual mechanisms for heating, air conditioning, water heating, and lighting are chosen, matching them to the loads expected from the design. Independent energy production using solar, wind or hydro power may also be included.

Integrating the site with the building and its technology can now be easily done with computer tools which give a better understanding of the energy implications of each design choice. A skilled designer or building technology specialist can learn to use these tools for simple buildings in a few hours, or they can hire an energy consultant to provide the service.

In the star diagram used in the case studies in this book, the length of the energy axis indicates how much energy conserving design was emphasized in the project, according to the author's assessment and the information provided by the design team or owner. If there is no energy emphasis shown on the diagram, the project is typical of conventional design, where energy is only considered as far as is necessary to meet basic code requirements. If the diagram shows a full energy emphasis, the project is considered highly advanced or "state of the art" and will typically use less than half the energy of a code compliant or standard building.

The Resource Conservation Emphasis

Material resources and water are solid forms of energy, so they are also environmental currency. As with energy, those who have resources are wealthy, and those who don't are poor. Squandering materials and water is also the tradition of the wealthy, while surviving with the minimum necessary for life is the experience of the poor. In the past two decades, access to good quality woods for construction has declined sharply through the entire world, and the cost has consequently increased. The cost of many other construction materials, such as metals, ceramics and plastics, has also increased. And the role of demolition and construction waste in our immense solid waste problem in urban areas has become apparent.

Our water sources are stretched to their limits in dry regions experiencing population growth. Many water sources are not renewable, and few new sources are likely to appear. Like energy conservation, material and water conservation require thinking differently and designing differently. Once again, wealthy societies are actually the best equipped to conserve.

35

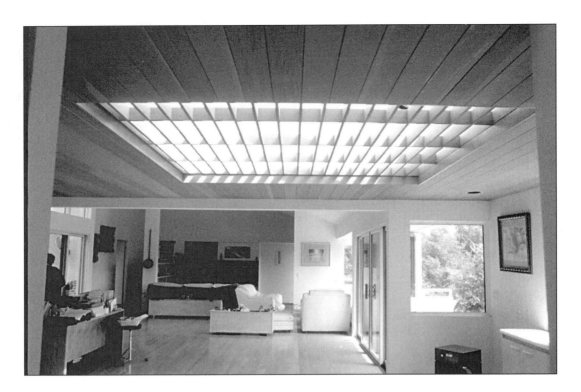

The energy efficient healthy home.

Resource-conserving building design and materials are the new frontier of the 1990s.

In the building sector, a materials conservation ethic has surfaced, and can be seen in the move toward using salvaged and recycled materials, resource efficient systems and, most recently, toward more compact and space-intensive building designs. Using these strategies, it is possible to provide quality housing, or other accommodation, using 25% to 50% less new materials than a conventional building requires.

Materials conservation in building design generally begins with an inventory of local resources, and those in standing buildings on the site. Salvaging all or parts of existing buildings is the first stage in conservation, followed by designing to reduce materials. Combining compact designs and optimum value engineering (advanced framing systems and materials which serve the same function with less raw material) can save perhaps 10% to 30% of the material used in a conventional design. Finding materials with recycled content and using locally available resources such as stone, earth, straw and wood is the next stage. Using manufactured products, such as engineered wood products, which use lower value resources or use resources more effectively, is the next stage. Waste reduction and recycling in demolition, construction and landscaping is the final stage.

Water conservation starts with an assessment of all the items requiring water in the building. A pool or spa is always a major water user, with little capacity for recycling because of the treatments required to maintain safe conditions. Extending the useful life of the water in the pool or spa with effective filters and treatment, and minimizing chemical additives by using ozone is usually the best that can be done.

The toilet is usually the next largest water user. Low-flush toilets, which save over half the water of conventional ones, are now standard and required by code in many areas. A composting toilet system uses no water at all, and is allowed by health codes in some regions.

Depending on climate and lot size, the garden may be the largest water user. But in most temperate climates, it is second to the toilets. In dry regions, using drought-resistant plants and ground cover to reduce evaporation are basic conservation strategies.

The shower and laundry are the next largest water users, followed by the sinks and dishwashers. Restrictive shower heads, tubs sculpted to fit the body and aerator faucets all save water. Laundry machines and dishwashers that use less water per cycle are now available.

The final water conservation strategy is on-site water collection, treatment and recycling. Rainwater can be collected for gardening and washing, and wastewater from bathing and the kitchen can be reused on the garden, depending on local codes and treatment requirements. Water treatment and reuse on-site, using constructed marshes, biological filters or aquatic greenhouses is also possible, if space and budget permit.

Material and water conservation are not just technical items to be considered after design; they can become a major organizer for design with exciting results. Salvaged building components and materials can be featured to make the most of their history and quality. And water collection, treatment and reuse can become an integral and beautiful part of the building and landscape.

In the star diagram used in the case studies in this book, the length of the resource axis indicates how much resource conserving design was emphasized in the project, according to the author's assessment and the information provided by the design team or owner. If there is no resource emphasis shown on the diagram, the project is typical of conventional design, where materials and water are used only according to preference, code requirements and budget. If the diagram shows a full resource emphasis, the project is considered to be highly advanced or "state of the art." It will typically be designed to use at least half salvaged, recycled-content or resource efficient materials and systems, produce less than half the landfilled waste of a typical project, and achieve water conservation which exceeds the code requirement by half.

BALANCING HEALTH, ENERGY AND RESOURCE EFFICIENCY

Health vs. Energy Efficiency

To a large degree, energy efficient design can also be healthy design. High-quality building envelopes and systems which provide good climate control, moisture control and comfort also tend to provide good control over air quality and sunlight and daylight conditions. In heating, cooling and ventilating systems, the most energy efficient combustion equipment is also the safest. The main conflicts between health and energy conservation occur around items such as ventilation rate, air filtration and electrical lighting type.

A higher mechanical ventilation capacity than the required minimum is often an emphasis in healthy design, so that the building can be "flushed" when needed, and odors and minor irritants can be thoroughly controlled. Fan-operated ventilation uses energy and, during heating and cooling periods, excess ventilation may cost substantially, because incoming air must be heated or cooled for comfort. Air filtration also uses energy. The most effective mechanical filters are also the most restrictive to air flow, and so require extra fan energy. Central scrubber filters for removing odors from intake air and recirculated air can add up to 200 watts to continuous electrical demand. Electronic filters use less energy, but cost more and capture only dust, not odors.

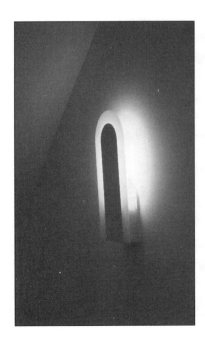

In lighting, the most energy efficient lamps are often not preferred for lighting quality, particularly for residential use. For example, the cool white fluorescent is the most efficient common lamp, but is the least desired for color balance and light quality. Fortunately, this situation is improving with new generation lamps, such as triphosphor-coated fluorescents and metal halides, generally used in commercial applications but with some residential uses as well. Electronic lamp ballasts now also offer freedom from flicker, better energy efficiency, and smaller magnetic fields. For residential use, compact fluorescent lamps are available in a good color range for warmth, and for rendering skin tones, and they use 25% to 35% of the

Energy efficient design can also be healthy design.

The new generation of compact fluorescent lamps allow elegant lighting while providing good color balance and excellent energy efficiency.

38

energy of a standard tungsten lamp for the same light output. Quartz lamps, or halogen lamps, are 15% to 30% more efficient than standard tungsten lamps, and provide a desirable light quality for display and reading use.

Health vs. Resource Efficiency

These two emphases are often in conflict, and only rarely complement one another. Many healthy materials, such as solid wood, concrete, masonry, ceramics, glass and metals require large amounts of raw materials and energy to manufacture and deliver. Also, many specialty products, such as low-toxicity finishes, are made only in one location, and so must be shipped long distances, and do not contribute to the local economy near the building site.

Engineered wood products made from low-quality or waste woods, such as chips, sawdust and fast-growing hardwoods are resource efficient but without exception are held together with adhesives, a source of air pollution. Some engineered wood products are over 10% glue, by weight.

Three factors can minimize the pollution potential of these products. First, if they are used outside the occupied space of the building, emissions are less likely to enter. Examples include outside wall and roof structural materials, which are excluded by an air/vapor barrier (used in cold climates). Second, the adhesive in materials rated for exterior use has very little formaldehyde offgassing potential, unlike interior adhesives which emit formaldehyde. Third, there are a number of interior products now made with chemically stabilized adhesive, exterior adhesive, or completely formaldehyde-free adhesive, all of which are safer than interior materials which are not stabilized.

Another conflict between resource efficiency and health is in the use of salvaged buildings and materials. It is very resource efficient to use salvaged buildings, but many are dirty and moisture damaged, and difficult to clean. They may contain asbestos and lead-based paint or plumbing. If paint stripping is required, it is a health risk and produces toxic waste. In some cases it is extraordinarily difficult and expensive to repair an old building to the point where it can be climate controlled and easily maintained.

In the case of water conservation, there are usually no conflicts with health, except that some water filtration systems used for health reasons may waste water by backwashing or flushing as they purify. Reverse osmosis water purifiers discharge about five times as much water to the drain as they treat, and if not equipped with an automatic standby valve, continue to waste water even when their tank is full and they are idle.

The main agreement between health and efficient use of resources are some plant fiber materials, earth materials and other natural materials used in healthy buildings. Many are from plentiful local and renewable resources, and their manufacture has a light environmental impact. Examples include straw and rammed earth, plaster and clay, jute, sisal and reed mats and fabric, and some wool and organic cotton products. The all-natural finishes made from linseed oil and earth pigments are also both healthy and resource efficient.

Resource vs. Energy Efficiency

The relationship between resource and energy efficiency seems initially to be one of conflict, but over the long term they are compatible. In order to achieve energy efficiency, there are often significant investments of materials and high-tech equipment which has a high initial environmental cost. Common examples are plastic insulations, high-performance windows, extra frame cavities for insulation and highly energy efficient furnaces and air conditioners. Alternative energy systems, such as solar hot water collectors, photovoltaic panels, wind or water turbines, and storage batteries also have high initial environmental cost from manufacturing. However, all of these energy efficiency and alternative energy features have a direct payback, in terms of fuels and electricity saved, and consequent air and water pollution and solid waste avoided.

Calculations of the payback on investments in materials and equipment used in residential energy efficiency and renewable energy projects shows that though they cost more, they are a sound environmental investment. Energy paybacks, comparing the energy invested in improvements with operating energy savings, for insulation, window improvements, and high efficiency heating and cooling equipment vary from a few months to a few years in a cold climate. Alternative energy systems are similar. Unfortunately, the dollar payback doesn't match the environmental payback very well. Some items, such as photovoltaic systems and solar water heaters, may take many years to pay back their initial dollar cost, depending on climate and specific situation. Some may never pay back completely during their useful lifetime. However, this is not really a failure of the idea or the technology; it is really a failure of our economic system, which does not reflect the true environmental cost of energy and commodities through their market price.

QUALITY AND COST

Healthy buildings usually cost more to build than unhealthy buildings. How much more depends on how rigorous the healthy approach is. Recent experience suggests that the healthy home which incorporates more

Resource-efficient buildings can also be energy efficient.

40

durable finishes, careful details and components to improve longevity and reduce maintenance, and some advanced approaches to heating and ventilation, may cost 10% to 15% more to build. However, the payback is difficult to judge, because many healthy building choices, such as durable finishes and high-quality heating and ventilation, lead to long-term operating savings and increased future value.

Is a healthy building a good investment? It is likely that something that makes environmental sense and provides a better setting for people today, will also make financial sense in the long term. Better quality buildings are likely to have an important edge in terms of reduced maintenance and operating cost, longer replacement cycles and improved user satisfaction and loyalty. Many people who have incorporated healthy building features are delighted, not only with the improved environment, but with the minimized cleaning requirements and freedom from regular repair and replacement of unhealthy items such as wall-to-wall carpet.

It is not a fair comparison to match a quality building with a minimum-cost builder's box. The increased initial cost of a healthy home can be more than offset by its durability and low maintenance, as well as its less tangible health and quality of life benefits. As well, in office, retail and school buildings, investments in quality and health reflect well on the judgment and leadership of owners, and in leased premises they can attract loyal tenants.

Quality vs. Quantity

One way to offset the increased initial cost of the healthy home is to scale down your size expectations and build smaller. How much space do you really need? How much space do you really use? How many bathrooms do you really need? People who live in apartments and compact townhouses learn to make maximum use of their space, and good design can make these small spaces functional and delightful.

A large home with many specialized rooms is not really much of a design challenge. It can be designed hastily, and put together carelessly, and will still function. But it is likely to always seem sloppy and awkward. In a smaller home, the challenge is to make everything function while still maintaining the feeling of generous space. A few keys to achieving this are:

- Always maintain one, major space in the design, usually multifunctional, such as a combined dining/living room. Resist the urge to divide everything as could be done in a larger home.
- Maintain generous daylight and both interior and exterior views. Large windows, carefully positioned skylights, and interior partitions

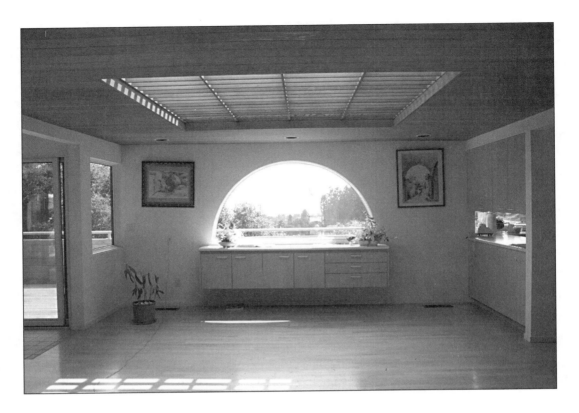

A healthy interior emphasizes space, daylight and view.

Healthy building practices can be applied to schools, clinics, offices and other buildings.

with openings or glass in them are helpful, where appropriate, to allow daylight in and maintain the long view.

- Do not let hallways and doors swallow up the space. Rooms must also serve as corridors, and doors should be used only where necessary for privacy.

Costs and payback in relation to the star diagram

Of the three types of emphasis, health, energy efficiency and resource efficiency, healthy building steps are likely to add the largest total cost increase to construction. Durable, dust- and volatile-free finishes are usually the largest cost items for healthy buildings. Ceramic tile and hardwood floors, for example, typically cost about two to three times as much as a mid-priced carpet. Carpet is often about 2% of total costs in conventional construction, which means that healthy floors can add about 4% to 6% to total cost. Other healthy finishes, such as traditional plaster and solid wood millwork require specialist trades and can be quite expensive.

Upgraded heating, air conditioning, ventilation and filtration systems are usually the next largest expense where health is emphasized. A radiant, hot water heating system, for example, may cost twice as much as a standard forced-air furnace. A hot water, fan-coil furnace with special filtration may be priced similarly. Either of these choices may add from 3% to 5% to total new construction costs. A ducted ventilation system may add 1.5% to 2% over a code minimum system, depending on whether heat recovery is used (usually based on climate) and whether or not the heating system is forced air. Air conditioning costs are usually unaffected by healthy building measures. If a heat pump is the heating source of choice, there is little additional cost for cooling.

A massive radiant heater (European style "tile oven") is a specific heating option which can be priced by a specialized supplier or stove builder. Tile or masonry heaters are expensive because their construction is quite labor intensive. There may also be code approval problems in some regions.

Other additional costs, such as a built-in vacuum with an outside vent, or a special water filtration system, are easily predicted because they are specific items from suppliers who usually have package prices.

As for paints, adhesives and sealants, the safer choices are usually similar in cost to conventional ones. Only special, all-natural paints and coatings are likely to cost more, because they are expensive to make, and many are imported. Fortunately the total cost of coatings and paints is rarely more than 0.5 % of total construction, and the labor to apply them is the same, so they have little net effect on total cost.

Some items, such as daylight design, weather sealing and special moisture control measures for wet climates, are difficult to predict because they are specific to each situation. Some will have no additional costs, while others will have modest costs. Special construction, such as timber, earth, straw and other alternative methods are labor intensive and may require special skills. In order to estimate costs for these it is necessary to have a design and speak with an experienced builder.

It is difficult to make a fair comparison between conventional construction and healthy construction because healthy construction incorporates the care, quality and attention to detail normally found only in high-end custom work. The results have paybacks which are apparent, but hard to measure. For example, the reduced maintenance, labor and costs of low-maintenance finishes and excellent dust control are tangible, but difficult to assign a dollar figure to. Other benefits, such as improved satisfaction and well-being, are nearly impossible to measure.

One direct and measurable payback is the savings from more durable materials, but these tend to occur over the long term. Typically maintenance savings, and savings on replacement of major materials such as roofing, siding and floor coverings, do not appear for 10 to 20 years. For example, consider a cement slate or concrete tile roof which costs three times as much as good-quality asphalt shingles. The asphalt shingles must be replaced in approximately 20 years, depending on climate and exposure. The slate or tile roof is almost certain to last over 50 years, and 75 or 100 years is not unlikely. Each replacement cycle of the asphalt shingle roof creates great disturbance for the occupants, and a lot of waste. A similar argument holds for hardwood or ceramic floors compared to carpet.

Energy efficiency steps are often also part of a healthy building, but it is hard to estimate the additional cost of energy efficient building elements items over conventional ones, because they are so case specific. However, a rough estimate of 15% to 20% additional for the building shell to obtain better insulation and windows is a good guide. Because the shell is less than half the cost of the building, the total impact on construction costs may be less than 10%. If energy efficiency and healthy building features are combined, however, the net result is not simply the sum of the two additional cost increments. Due to the overlap of some healthy features and energy efficient features, the combined cost is less. Common examples of energy efficiency steps are passive solar design, high-quality insulation and windows, and draft sealing to improve comfort, moisture control and ventilation control. Energy efficient, fuel-burning furnaces and water heaters are also, coincidentally, very unlikely to contaminate the home with combustion gases.

The important cost difference between energy efficiency and healthy building features is that energy efficiency features have a measurable payback in terms of reduced energy bills. The payback period is dependent on the particular feature, the climate and utility costs, but it is fair to say that extra insulation and draft sealing pay back within a few years in a heating or air conditioning climate. The more severe the climate, the faster the payback. Some features, such as advanced windows, solar hot water heaters, and photovoltaic panels, may take many years to show a savings, as noted earlier. However, payback is often not the main reason energy efficiency is included in new construction or remodeling. An energy efficient building is usually a very comfortable and durable building, with reduced maintenance needs.

Resource efficiency steps include designing smaller buildings with more efficient use of space, the use of durable, resource efficient and recycled materials, and water conservation. Many of these steps actually cost less, particularly if the amount of material used is less. Only some of the

There are many rewards for healthy construction, some tangible and some difficult to measure.

more durable materials, and some materials with recycled content tend to cost more. There are also immediate paybacks for some resource efficient materials. For example, wood "I Joists" or "open web" joists are very resource efficient for floor and roof framing because they are made from small pieces of wood, and do not require the large trees necessary for 2x10 and 2x12 lumber. They usually cost a little more, but they make it possible to run ventilation, heating ducts, plumbing and wiring through the members much more easily than with solid wood. And they do not shrink or warp, so there are fewer problems after construction. These two advantages alone are usually worth more than the small additional cost.

Water conserving plumbing fixtures are very simple, and usually cost no more than inefficient types when new. They may be available for free or for a very small cost in some cities which have incentive programs to replace old fixtures. Even if you pay the full replacement cost for low-flush toilets, the payback may be as little as one year, depending on your water rates.

One way to reduce costs and to get involved with the building is to do some of the labor yourself, if you are available and capable. Almost anyone can do jobs such as handling soil, cleanup, and some painting and landscaping tasks.

CHAPTER 5

The Healthy Remodel

Remodeling is a popular and growing trend. Many people wish to improve their homes, but don't have the money to rebuild entirely. Unfortunately, not all homes are good candidates for remodeling, especially from a healthy building standpoint. Major problems, such as asbestos and lead removal, and earthquake upgrading, can make remodeling prohibitively complicated and expensive. A building with serious undesirable features, such as a bad floor plan, very small rooms or poor siting on the lot, may also not be worth remodeling.

Remodeling a home or office with good features is usually more resource efficient than demolishing it and starting again, particularly if the building is in sound condition and the remodel takes advantage of the building's merits. Compared with new construction, a typical total residential remodel, including new walls, flooring, plumbing, wiring, painting and roofing saves about 30 cubic yards of landfill (2 1/2 tandem truckloads). It saves enough energy in the production of new materials ("embodied energy") to operate the house for over two years. An efficient and well-executed remodel may also save the owners as much as half the cost of new construction.

Professional advice is invaluable to assess whether or not a building is suitable for remodeling, and to work out a good design. Remodeling specifically for health, rather than esthetic or other reasons, is an even more specialized task which makes a professional assessment of the existing building imperative. Some of the most important questions to consider before beginning a healthy building remodel are:

- Is the site appropriate for the health goals?
- Is it free from excessive noise, air pollution and soil pollution?
- Are the wind, daylight and sunlight exposure and view desirable?
- Are the plants around the building minimal pollen producers and well tolerated?

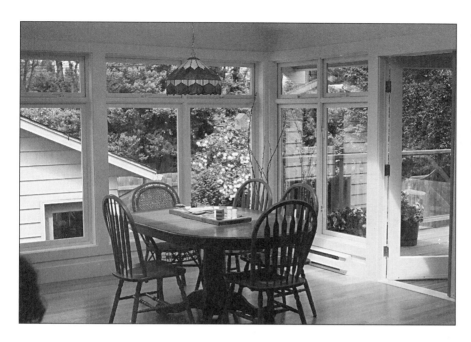

An older home with generous rooms, good light, view and pleasant surroundings may be a good candidate for a healthy remodel.

- Is the building sound and dry, and free from any recent history of leaks, smokers, poor cleaning and maintenance, and pesticide treatments?
- Has the building been free of termites, rodents, cockroaches, ants and other pests?
- Have any significant lead or asbestos problems in the building been remedied?
- Are the heating, air conditioning and ventilation systems the type you want and, if not, are they practical to replace?

If the answers to these, and some of the usual important questions about location, esthetic appeal, and cost are promising, then the building may be worth investigating further, and some design and costing done.

WHAT TO LOOK FOR

The best candidates for a healthy remodel are generally between approximately 5 and 20 years old. A building over five years old generally has very little offgassing from original construction materials such as carpets, vinyl floors and underlay, decorative plywoods, furniture and cabinets, doors and paints. The major indoor air pollution sources in a house this age come from occupants, activities and poor maintainence: soiled carpets, dirty

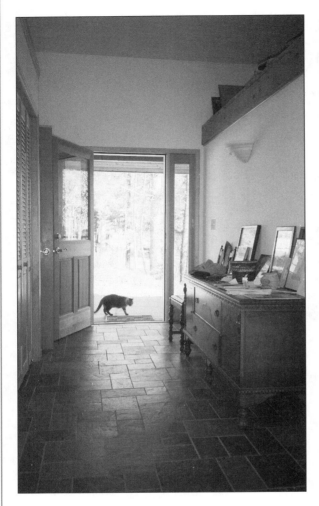

Durable floor finishes help to make a home a good candidate for a healthy remodel.

walls and ceilings, dusty air ducts, kitchen grease, odors from smokers and so on. A home this age is also less likely to have serious accumulations of dust in cavities, rotted framing, cracked plaster and sagging foundations than one over 20 years old.

Houses over 20 years old may have serious dust accumulation and stale odors everywhere. Walls and ceilings may be filled with dust which will be disturbed during remodeling work, and they are also likely to have deteriorating plaster and woodwork and peeling paint which will require repair and replacement. Older houses may also have dry rot, or have been treated extensively for pests. Buildings over about 30 years old which have not been remodeled are usually the most expensive and difficult to remodel because they tend to have very poor insulation and draft sealing, poor windows and doors, and need to have their original plumbing, heating and wiring replaced, and possibly air conditioning added. These are also the most likely to contain asbestos and lead.

Slab construction with radiant heat or hot water convectors is another important feature in a healthy remodel candidate. Buildings on a slab tend to be more dust- and mildew-free, and have fewer soil gas and moisture problems than buildings with basements and crawl spaces. The advantage of radiant heat or hot water convectors (also called hydronic heat) is that, unlike conventional furnaces, this type of heat does not stir up dust, or overheat dust, causing it to produce odors and fine carbon particles (sometimes called fried dust). The disadvantage of these systems is that, in a very cold or warm climate in which the building will be closed up for much of the year for heating or cooling, it will usually be necessary to add a ventilation, and possibly an air filtration system as well. This system will require some ducts since there will usually be none. See Heating and Air Conditioning in chapter 8 for more detail.

Houses suitable for healthy remodeling should also have durable and dust-free interior finishes, such as hardwood, ceramic tile and plaster.

Hardwood and ceramic floors help with dust control, have low volatile emissions and require little maintenance. Wood floors in need of refinishing are still an advantage, so long as the building can be vacated for at least two weeks for the new finish to cure. It will also be necessary to do a complete dust cleanup after sanding. Traditional plaster interiors may be better than gypsum wallboard because their surface is very hard and nonporous, but they must be in good condition and free of major cracks.

Old wood wall paneling may not be an advantage because often it has been exposed to dampness and dust, and is not fully sealed and finished the way a wood floor is. It may also have a lot of cracks and joints, making it difficult to clean. Wood paneling may become "stale" after many years from absorbed household odors. This is particularly true of softwoods such as fir and pine.

Look for permanent, well-maintained roofing and siding. The building should have a well-designed, constructed and maintained outer shell with little need for major modifications or repairs. Changing windows and reroofing are two of the most expensive exterior repairs in remodeling. Brick faced buildings, and those with tile or slate roofs have major advantages because they are very permanent and low maintenance. However, they must be in good condition; they are very expensive to repair if poorly maintained.

WHAT TO AVOID

A healthy remodeling project may not be worthwhile if the home's problems are too many or too serious. For instance, extensive, concealed rot or insect damage, especially in bathrooms, attics, and around foundations are complicated and expensive to fix. Extensive moisture damage is certain to cause fungus contamination which is very difficult to completely remove. Severe insect damage may already have been treated with a toxic, residual pesticide and if there is chronic infestation, it may be difficult to completely prevent in future without pesticides because buildings which have not been built to keep insects out are often very difficult to seal later.

Cracks and chronic leaks around foundations make healthy remodels difficult. Dampness and cracks usually lead to fungus growth and often indicate paths for soil gas entry. If the foundation has serious drainage problems, it is usually necessary to excavate around it to repair it from the outside. For a full basement, this is very expensive and disruptive for occupants and gardens.

A raised wood basement floor is also a serious problem. If a wood floor has been placed on an old concrete basement slab, using wood strips (called sleepers) resting on the concrete, it is almost certain to have a trapped air space between the concrete and the wood which encourages moisture, rot and insects. If the floor has been in place for several years, it is likely to have fungus contamination in the cavity space. Only chemically treated wood or extremely rot-resistant wood can withstand these conditions. In a very dry climate, rot and fungus are a smaller problem, and can be prevented in new construction by insulating and moisture sealing the base under the slab. The slab can also be heated.

If there is an old coal bin in the basement or there has been oil- or coal-burning equipment in the building, there are often areas where the building or the surrounding soil has been contaminated. Oil residue in soil, concrete or wood is very difficult to clean up. The soil usually has to be removed and disposed of.

An attached garage or old hobby space can be a serious health and fire risk if it has been used for fuel and oil storage, automotive repair, garden chemical or other chemical storage. Particularly in older buildings, the common wall and door between the garage and living space are difficult to seal. Heating or air conditioning ducts which are part of ceilings or floors and not lined with sheet metal or, worst of all, buried in concrete, are nearly impossible to maintain. If they have rough surfaces, wood sides, inside insulation or obstructions, they will trap dust, odors and allergenic particles and contaminate the air stream. The best solution is to remove all these and replace them with new sheet metal ducts which are fully accessible for cleaning.

Note: Adding air conditioning during a remodel will require ensuring that insulation, windows and ductwork (in a central, forced-air system) are all adequate. For smaller remodels, a "split system" unit is useful for a single room or small suite. See Heating and Air Conditioning in chapter 8.

If the building was insulated after it was built, the walls and ceilings are probably filled with a loosefill insulation which was blown or poured into the cavities. Retrofitted insulation done decades ago may be vermiculite or perlite (expanded minerals) or any number of other materials such as shredded wood, bark or straw. More recent retrofits are likely to be cellulose (shredded newsprint) or chopped fiberglass or mineral wool. All of these materials are hazardous to some degree, or highly allergenic, if they leak into the building, which they are very likely to do in older construction, especially during remodeling. In many buildings there is no barrier to prevent dust, fibers and odors from wall and ceiling cavities from entering the living spaces. The expanded minerals and chopped glass or mineral fiber

Remodeling without extra precautions may seriously aggravate dust problems from concealed sources.

present the highest risk of lung injury. The cellulose, wood and plant materials are very irritating, especially the more recent products which contain fire retardants.

If remodeling a building with loosefill insulation, it is safest to entirely remove the insulation from all affected areas before any demolition is done. This should be done with a shovel and commercial vacuum. All potential paths where insulation can enter the building should also be sealed in those areas not remodeled. See chapter 10 for more detail on healthy construction management.

Moisture Control

Chronic moisture indoors is one of the leading causes of poor indoor air and is a major concern in a healthy remodel. Moist surfaces will support fungi such as mildew, which produce stale and musty odors. They also release tiny particles which can cause mild to severe allergic reactions. The musty odor from a mildewed surface is not just a nuisance, it is an indicator of volatile chemicals produced by the fungi, some of which are quite toxic. The most common moisture problems are:

- leaky basements and crawl spaces
- inadequately ventilated, dehumidified or heated basements and crawl spaces
- carpets and wood floors placed on concrete basement slabs
- poorly ventilated bathrooms, laundries and kitchens
- poor-quality windows that sweat
- areas with poor insulation causing cold spots on walls and ceilings
- roof and wall leaks causing damp framing, insulation and inside surfaces
- poorly maintained air conditioners, dehumidifiers, and humidifiers
- a heated building with substantial air leakage into insulated spaces in a cold climate (causing concealed moisture)
- an air conditioned building with substantial air infiltration in a humid climate

If any of these problems are apparent, repairing them should be a high priority in your remodel.

Before purchasing a building for remodeling, or when planning a substantial remodel of one you already own, it is best to hire a qualified home inspector to do a complete survey report on the condition of the building. The inspector should be told that health conditions are particularly important. If you plan to hire an architect or experienced designer, their first

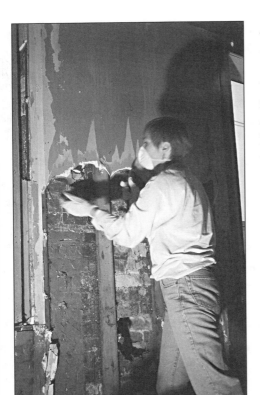

Always expect surprises when remodeling an older building.

task should be to undertake this assessment. The modest cost of the inspection will be recovered several times over if the remodel goes ahead, because the knowledge is essential for planning and budgeting. If the inspection report causes you to decide against the purchase or remodel, it is a small price to pay for the avoided grief.

PROTECTING OCCUPANTS DURING REMODELING

Many homes are occupied during remodeling, and occupants suffer nuisance and health risks from exposure to dusts, solvents, noise and various pollutants. Dust problems may last several months after construction is complete. The following precautions will help to make your remodel healthier and easier to tolerate:

If possible, vacate when you remodel.

- Vacate the home during the entire demolition and construction period, if possible. Furniture and clothing should be moved out, or relocated to an area which will not be disturbed and covered with plastic sheets. If this is done, some of the following precautions are less critical.
- Isolate the construction area before demolition, using tarps taped to walls and ceilings. Close off all doors and other openings to areas which are not being remodeled. The heating, air conditioning and ventilation systems should be shut off in the work areas, and grilles covered with foil or plastic. If possible, these systems should not be used during demolition and dusty finishing work. If a forced-air furnace must be used during remodeling to heat the area not being renovated, be sure that the airflow is sufficient for normal operation after closing off the grilles to the work area.
- If a roof will be removed, a heavy tarp or temporary floor should be placed over the ceiling joists below it to reduce the dust and debris which fall through into the home.

- A no-smoking policy on the jobsite will prevent odors which may cause complaints. Ashes and butts are also a cleaning problem. Smoking should be restricted to outdoors, well away from the building.

- Ventilate temporarily with portable fans, and open windows in the renovation area. This is especially important during painting and when adhesives must be used. A small fan in a window can also be used to pressurize the area not being renovated, to reduce migration of dust and odors from the renovation area.

- Heat temporarily for drywall work in cool weather, and to cure paints, adhesives, caulkings and other materials that need to set or dry. It will also help prevent moisture damage if wet materials have been brought in, or if there has been any water leakage. Avoid unvented propane heaters; they produce a great deal of moisture which slows drying. Electric construction heaters are best.

- Clean up after the work is complete. This should include not only vacuuming, mopping and glass cleaning, but also dusting of walls and ceilings with a damp cloth or mop, and cleaning of furnace ducts. If there is no built-in vacuum, a portable vacuum with a HEPA (high-efficiency particulate arrestance) filter is effective for final dust cleanup. Avoid ammonia and chlorine cleansers if possible, and highly scented products. The safest cleansers are vinegar, baking soda, washing soda (sodium carbonate) and TSP (trisodium phosphate).

CHAPTER 6

Site Selection, Site Planning and Architectural Design

Choosing a location, and planning the site and the design of your house have an important effect on how the house responds to the three points of concern: health, energy, and resource efficiency. This chapter introduces issues of planning and design, focusing on basic design strategies that incorporate all three concerns.

SITE SELECTION

For fortified towns the following general principles are to be observed. First comes the choice of a very healthy site. Such a site will be high, neither misty nor frosty, and in a climate neither hot nor cold, but temperate; further, without marshes in the neighborhood. For when the morning breezes blow toward the town at sunrise, if they bring with them mists from marshes and, mingled with the mist, the poisonous breath of the creatures of the marshes to be wafted into the bodies of the inhabitants, they will make the site unhealthy. —VITRUVIUS

Location has as much impact as any other decision on the environmental attributes of a home. This is true whether you are drawn toward urban or rural life, a choice endlessly debated on environmental grounds. Urban life, at its best, is by far the most energy and resource efficient choice. At its worst, urban living cuts us off from the ecological impact of our actions, undermining its potential advantages. Rural life at its best is nurturing for the land as well as the psyche. At its worst it destroys the very qualities that make it attractive, turning farmland into sprawl. Both urban and rural sites can be healthy, stimulating environments but both have special qualities and shortcomings which you need to identify, either before you buy, or as you work to heal and protect the place you already own.

The general issues of site selection are the same in the city or the country, but the specifics will vary from one site to the next. Your goal should be to insure that the location you are considering does not present any unusual environmental hazards: the air should be relatively clean and fresh; the soil should not hide hazardous residues from previous uses; the ground water should be safe, particularly if you are depending on it; and sources of stress, such as noise, should be manageable. The environmental attributes of a good site are universal: the dwelling should have some direct exposure to the sun and the potential for good, natural ventilation; the site and its surroundings should be relatively well drained. Sites exposed to odors from industry or agriculture often produce complaints and should be avoided even if the odors are not specifically hazardous. Radon emissions and other gases from the soil are a possible natural hazard that should be evaluated and designed for if present (see the Table of Common Air Pollutants in chapter 3 and the foundation details in the 79 Best Healthy Building Solutions). The presence of high-tension power lines, cellular telephone relay stations or other radio, television or microwave installations are also a specific concern (see Electromagnetic Fields in chapter 3).

In evaluating any location, you should attempt to answer several fundamental questions. The first question is whether the property itself is healthy or can be made healthy. The second question is whether the surrounding area is acceptable and you understand its uses throughout the year. You don't want to buy a house in the middle of winter and wake up months later to gridlock outside your front door caused by opening day at the stadium or racetrack down the street. The final and most difficult task is to imagine the area 5 or 25 years into the future, and ask yourself whether the qualities that make it desirable now will be enhanced or diminished by time.

When considering the placement of your home, recognize that you yourself are participating in the process of change, bringing both positive and negative impacts to the area. Changes may be beyond your control, but are not beyond prediction. Are there major developments planned that will alter the traffic patterns on your street, for example? Beyond the question of growth, look into the future to the possibility of a catastrophic accident occurring in your back yard. Much of California lives with the likelihood of earthquakes and brush fires. Other communities have been built and rebuilt in the paths of rivers and hurricanes. Others live with the risk of a chemical spill from a local industry, or even a local rail line serving distant customers and carrying hazardous cargo. These risks can be avoided, but we often choose not to, for whatever reason, and so we have to work to minimize the threat of both accident and overdevelopment through awareness and design.

Pollution Mapping

When investigating a site, think of yourself as an amateur mapmaker, charting the territory in which you live. Use an actual map, such as a city street map, as a starting point in evaluating your site, because it forces you to see your site from the point of view of a bird, erasing the boundaries that we draw around our experience. A factory on the opposite bank of a river, for example, might seem far away because it is hard to get to, but seeing its distance as the crow flies may reveal it to be uncomfortably close. There is no easy answer as to how large an area you need to be concerned about. Start by drawing a circle one mile in all directions and get to know this neighborhood well.

There is no question that urban air quality is often less than pristine. Air quality varies from one city to the next and from one location to the next, depending on geography and weather patterns, as well as on concentrated and dispersed sources of pollutants. You can probably find out the overall conditions of your city easily. Most newspapers print air pollution indexes that monitor local conditions, and the EPA publishes recommended maximum exposures for urban air pollution. If your experience tells you that the city as a whole is livable, your job is to be wary of more localized problems. In rural areas, chemical agriculture, major highways, rail lines and airports are typical items to identify and map. Large industries such as mines, mills and smelters may also be present, as well as polluted rivers and lakes.

Sources of air pollution can be roughly categorized on your map as "point sources," "line sources," and "dispersed sources." Point sources are large, identifiable polluters, such as industries or municipal power stations. Line sources are major roadways, which generate localized ribbons of particulate-laden air from tailpipe emissions, disintegrating tires and brakes, and dirt kicked up by heavy traffic. Dispersed sources are emissions from small-scale commercial activities, such as gas stations, dry cleaners and commercial kitchens, as well as residential sources such as gas lawn mowers and barbecues. Recent studies show, for example, that a third of the ozone pollution alert days in the Lake Michigan basin are on weekends, when a quarter of emission sources are not industries and commuters, but lawn mowers and pleasure boats.

Topography and wind patterns are as important as pollution sources, and may present simple clues in evaluating your site. Industrial sites are

Mapping the site and local region can be helpful when choosing a location.

56

often located in low-lying river valleys. This geographic feature often acts as a basin for foul air, making the air quality in one area distinctly different than in another. The surrounding landscape may also affect how wind moves, and hence which areas are cleaner and clearer than others. These distinctions are often subtle and go unnoticed unless you stop to think about them.

Point sources are the most highly regulated type of air pollution. If you have questions about the air quality of the region as a whole, or about a specific industry or another point source of air pollution, information can be obtained from local government agencies or from local environmental organizations. One place to start is the state air quality enforcement agency or provincial health department listed in the phone book. The agency will be able to provide a list of local agencies, where you can review industry permits and complaints on file for a given point source. Another source of technical information in the United States is the Toxic Release Inventory (TRI) maintained by the Environmental Protection Agency. The TRI lists emissions of major pollution sources by zip code and is available through your state EPA office or on the Internet [www.epa.gov/enviro].

In the book *The Granite Garden: Urban Nature and Human Design* Anne Whinston Spirn describes the line source pollution created by automobiles and the urban design strategies that can control its impact. The air quality of such corridors can become quite bad, especially if the street is set within a continuous canyon of high buildings that restrict natural air flow patterns. The book recommends a buffer zone of 50 meters (164 feet) from the edge of a major arterial road to any residential use, planted with a dense wall of street trees and ground cover to act as a filter and noise buffer. If you are considering a site on a major street you may want to approach the choice with caution. At minimum, visit the area at various times of day to understand the actual traffic loads. Spend enough time there to test your own level of comfort. For more information, contact your metropolitan planning organization, which is responsible for transportation modeling. It will be able to provide traffic counts, and more importantly, information on congestion, which produces greater levels of both noise and localized pollution. Finally, it should be able to provide projections of future growth and information on planned road expansion.

Less obvious, and of particular concern, are the little-regulated dispersed sources of pollution. Sites immediately adjacent to potential sources of fumes such as auto body shops or dry cleaners, should be avoided altogether or designed for with special care. Loading docks where diesel trucks idle are a particular problem.

A final source of local air pollution associated with environmental health problems is pesticide use. This issue cuts across the urban/rural divide. On one hand, the use of pesticides by individual urban and suburban homeowners is less regulated than larger scale applications, with the result that the amounts applied are often much more concentrated. On the other hand, it is much more likely in a rural agricultural setting that the pesticide will be applied from the air and that you will be dependent on ground or well water carrying residual pesticides.

In both urban and rural locations, the type and extent of pesticide use is dependent on the climate and other local conditions. In the hot and humid southern United States, for example, termites are a major problem for home owners and the casual use of insecticides inside the home has led to serious health complaints. From Canada to Mexico, mosquito control is also connected to pesticide use. Try to develop a sense of your area's local problems and practices. Are the lawns of your suburban neighborhood immaculately manicured, and if so what sorts of steps do people take to keep them that way? How is the urban park near you maintained? Are your rural roadway shoulders or power line cuts regularly defoliated by the County Works department or local utility?

This traditional lawn is unusual in that it is maintained without pesticides, using only organic fertilizers.

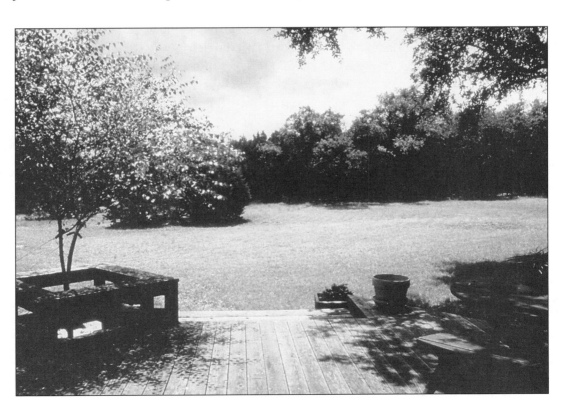

Local attitudes toward pesticides vary greatly. Many states have uniform, if limited, programs creating registries of sites where pesticides are used, posting signs on treated lawns and certifying professional applicators. Often, city parks boards are more responsive than private entities to concern over pesticide use, while institutions such as hospitals and schools, ironically, tend to be heavy users.

In general, open lands managed in a more or less natural state are a good sign, as are dandelions in a lawn. A few phone calls to the local government agencies in charge of overseeing environmental issues, or to your local Sierra Club or similar environmental organization should help you determine whether there is reason for concern, and if efforts to restrict local pesticide use are underway.

In both urban and rural settings, learning the history of the site is important in order to avoid assuming responsibility for an unhealthy legacy such as buried waste or contaminated soil. Not all contamination is equally troubling. It is likely that any older, painted house will have some amount of lead contamination indoors and in the soil immediately adjacent to it, for example. The degree to which outdoor lead is a concern is dependent on whether you will have children in the yard, where you locate your garden, and on the design of the house so that potentially lead-contaminated mud is not tracked in. An older house with lead paint on the exterior will often have lead paint on the interior as well, which is a more serious concern. Evidence of illegal waste dumping on a rural site, or an underground storage tank from an old gas station or fuel oil storage may be a much more serious concern, partly because remediation is likely to be more costly, and partly because responsibility for cleanup is likely to have complicated legal implications.

If the site has not always been residential, or if it is on the border of non-residential land, you should find out what the former uses were and who the neighbors were. A title search will turn up some of this information. Current and historical aerial photography can be obtained from either the local government or a private map company, and can help to reveal previous uses. If you feel there is real reason for concern, an environmental consultant can be hired to do further investigative research and analysis. Remember that the property may have changed hands many times and the uses may also have changed several times. For example, many residential areas once had manufacturing or repair shops which handled oil, paints and solvents, and produced waste. Many smaller problems can be remediated, and often this will be required by law. Any purchase agreement should be contingent on the property receiving a clean bill of health.

Many severely hypersensitive people choose to live in rural settings if they can, removing themselves from the threat of polluted air to the greatest degree possible. Unfortunately, rural air quality cannot be assumed to be any better than urban air quality. In the Midwest, for example, a major study on ozone pollution has found the highest sustained levels of hazardous ozone exposure occur on the rural northwestern shores of Lake Michigan, hundreds of miles downwind from the industrial sources. Maps showing areas of unacceptably high ozone levels are of limited value, as the monitoring done is far from comprehensive. Again, if there is any reason for concern, talking to health officials in your area will provide you with locally relevant information.

The other air quality concern in rural sites is the impact of agricultural practices. Agricultural pesticide exposure should be avoided, and some people have difficulty breathing if and when land is periodically burned for clearing. For these reasons, the most desirable therapeutic landscapes for the environmentally hypersensitive are, in many ways, the most barren landscapes. The Hill Country of central Texas for example, where several healthy houses discussed in this book are located, is a scrub landscape that is both beautiful and agriculturally unproductive.

A separate but related issue is whether a particular landscape will trigger any conventional allergies that you might have. Some individuals even react to the terpenes present in various softwoods, such as pine. While it may not be possible to completely eliminate these irritants from your surroundings, you can minimize their impact by avoidance. Remember when visiting a site that allergies are often seasonal and may not be expressed at a given time of year.

Bruce Small, a healthy housing consultant outside Toronto, Ontario, offers a perspective on the often difficult trade-offs that health constraints place on finding the location of your dreams. Unable to find nonagricultural land to build on near Toronto, Bruce and his wife settled for a windswept knoll in the farming country outside of the city. They reasoned that if they were going to live in an agricultural setting, a windy location would ensure that any pesticide exposure would be brief and the air would generally be fresh. Bruce further reasoned that given his wife's and his own particular allergies and hypersensitivities, the medical establishment had more to offer in the way of conventional allergy medications than cures for chemical sensitivities. They chose to live with what they could treat and to avoid what they couldn't. This is ultimately the balance that we must strike as we weigh the complicated factors involved in choosing a place to live.

Pesticides may be a serious problem in both urban and rural locations.

SITE PLANNING

Site planning involves the design of the entire site and consideration of its impact on adjacent sites, such as the control of storm water runoff, or protecting a neighbor's view, or exposure to the sun. The main goal might be to "do no environmental harm," which may mean declining to develop a given parcel of land altogether. Once an appropriate site has been selected, you should work to save what is best about a place and build where your actions will have a positive impact.

In terms of health, proper site planning and design can partly mitigate environmental problems such as local air or noise pollution. Both can be reduced by creating buffers, and by zoning the site as a series of layers, from the most affected to the most protected. Trees and ground vegetation help capture airborne particulates; dense plantings such as deep hedges can also reduce noise, especially when located close to the source. Earth berms are often used around highways to create acoustic barriers that absorb as well as deflect traffic noise. Landscape features such as moving water or the rustling leaves of a tree near the dwelling can also be used to mask background noises.

Another potential health problem at a site is poor drainage, dense shade and still air. These attributes can create a beautiful marshland, supporting birds, insects and fish, but they can also create unhealthy conditions by providing habitat for molds and biting insects such as mosquitoes. Mosquitoes are an obvious nuisance and invite the use of pesticides, if not by you, then by your neighbor. High mold counts outdoors may be a mild nuisance or a severe health risk, depending on mold types and individual sensitivity.

Much of the technical information presented in this book deals with designing the structure and heating and ventilating systems of your home so that pesticides are not necessary and molds do not grow. The same logic applies to landscaping. Poorly drained soil can be avoided or altered by engineering the site for better drainage, if doing so does not conflict with wetland preservation. Often the simplest strategy is to clear the site immediately adjacent to the house, allowing the sun and air to dry the ground. In the case of the Oetzel House (see Case Study 7), the brush has been cleared away from the house, creating a conventional lawn that is maintained with organic fertilizers. At the Pitman House (see Case Study 8), the natural landscape is preserved and featured. The house is located at the edge of a natural clearing so that the southern frontal exposure looks into the trees while the potentially damp north side is open to the clearing.

The lawn of the Oetzel House was developed to control the mosquito population without using pesticides, by drying up their habitat. There is a growing body of literature on integrated pest management, permaculture and natural landscaping that describes landscaping and gardening strategies that work with rather than against natural processes by building the conditions for self-protecting and self-maintaining landscapes.

ARCHITECTURAL DESIGN

Climate-Responsive Design

A screened or glass enclosed porch can maintain a connection to the site in the healthy home, while protecting occupants from insects and extreme climate conditions.

The case studies in this book illustrate healthy housing constructed in a variety of climates. Note the differences in design approach between them based on their locations. The demonstration house in Toronto, Ontario is necessarily different from the log cabin house in Texas. The mild Texas climate allows the log house to transform itself into a huge screened porch, sheltered but only minimally enclosed. The Toronto house combines thick, well-insulated walls with large areas of glass facing the sun, to capture and retain heat. These differences in the ways the buildings interact with their respective climates determine the types of construction materials used, the choice of heating and cooling systems, and even the physical arrangement

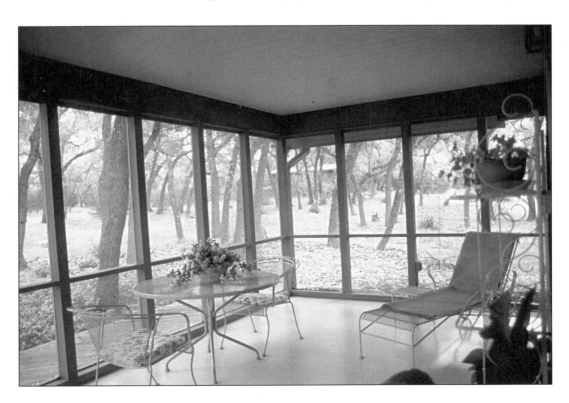

of the rooms as they affect indoor air quality. The climate in which you are building has an impact not only on the resource and energy efficiency points of concern, but on the health one as well.

There are four basic climate zones in North America presenting distinctly different conditions to design for: hot and humid, hot and dry, temperate, and cold.

The Gulf Coast from Miami, Florida to Houston, Texas typifies a hot and humid climate. High temperatures combine with high humidity to create a setting with very little daily variation in temperature, and few ways to remove excess heat and humidity without resorting to mechanical air conditioning. Such a climate poses a challenge for both energy and health concerns. This climate is, in some ways, the most difficult to design for, and the least well studied. Also, while it presents less than ideal conditions for human habitation, the combination of heat and humidity helps many other life forms to thrive. This leads to high use of pesticides, and makes mold and mildew substantial indoor air quality concerns.

The American Southwest, in particular Arizona and New Mexico, typifies a hot and dry climate. Without the stabilizing presence of water in the atmosphere, a hot, dry climate is marked by extreme temperature swings between day and night, regardless of the season. Even in summer, when daytime temperatures are above 100°F (38°C), night temperatures may plummet to the low 60s (16°C). These swings can be harnessed by climate-responsive architecture, building on the timeless logic of the region's adobe architecture, which delays the transfer of heat from the outside in just long enough to keep the internal temperatures comfortable and relatively constant. The lack of biological activity in a hot, dry climate is advantageous because it produces little mold growth and insect pests. Much of this region does not support agriculture, which makes it attractive for people who are seeking exceptionally pristine air. But the dryness itself can lead to respiratory problems for some people. Dryness, however, is easily adjusted by evaporative humidification, which also aids cooling.

The temperate zone is a catch-all of climate conditions that demand some heating in the winter and often cooling in the summer. The temperate zone blankets most of the continental United States, encompassing a huge variety of local climate conditions. For example the climate of coastal Oregon, Washington State and southern British Columbia is tempered by the Pacific Ocean and ranges from 20°F (−8°C) to 75°F (24°C) typically. The variety and variability of temperate climates suggests a wide range of possible design strategies. Solar energy capture, good thermal insulation, and natural ventilation are all potentially useful and important. The specifics of

63

the particular climate and exposure must be identified to achieve the most efficient design, but many solutions can be made to work well.

Finally, the cold climate zone blankets most of Canada, except for the Pacific coast, and sweeps down across the upper plains states of the United States. With long, cold winters and short, hot summers, often with high humidity, this climate is demanding but unambiguous. Passive design principles, such as capturing solar energy, plays a secondary role to insulation to prevent heat loss. The priority of the healthy house designer is to conserve heat without compromising indoor air quality, leading to the combination of superinsulated construction and carefully designed mechanical ventilation, a strategy that this book details. The Toronto Healthy House illustrates an aggressive combination of energy, health and resource conservation strategies appropriate for its cold climate.

Climate, Health and Building Form

Traditional house styles from each climate zone can provide clues about the most efficient building form for the region. Architecture for the hot and humid southern states is best expressed in the plantation house, an airy structure with high ceilings and deep porches. This form was designed to create a shaded outdoor living space, elevated above damp ground to capture breezes. Desert architecture moves in the opposite direction, digging into the ground for shelter, with solid walls facing the sun for warmth, while offering only limited openings to control glare and provide a cool, dark refuge from the intense heat of the summer day. Temperate dwellings provide shelter from rain and snow with a variety of roof forms but are fairly unconstrained in plan. Seasonal variation in climatic conditions is expressed by spaces such as porches with storm windows. Architecture for a cold climate is characterized by a compact form, minimizing the exposed surface of the dwelling, and historically gathering rooms around a central source of heat, such as a hearth.

The traditional logic of the climate zone can be seen in many of the case study houses. There is generally a relationship between the compactness of the plan and the severity of the climate, though economics also play a role. Climate-responsive design also requires an awareness of the sun's position in the sky, daily and seasonally, with thought given to capturing and controlling the sun on the southern exposure. This often leads to elongation of the house along the east/west axis, which expands the southern wall and minimizes the more difficult to control eastern and western exposures.

Individual rooms are also often located to take advantage of the sun's movement. Kitchens are typically to the east for early morning sun, family

There are four basic climate zones in North America presenting distinctly different conditions to design for: hot and humid, hot and dry, temperate, and cold.

areas to the south for warmth, and service areas such as garages, toilets and storage placed to the north. The organization of rooms by various attributes is referred to as the "plan zoning," a concept that has particular resonance in healthy house design.

Just as the plan of a house itself is zoned, the landscape around a house is a series of layers or zones. These layers can be used to help heat or cool the house. The design can alternately admit, filter or block the sun, wind and precipitation in order to create sunny, sheltered spaces that are comfortable when it is cold outside or shady, breezy spaces that are refreshingly cool when it is hot. These seasonal spaces are relatively inexpensive to build, and even in the city the air outside is likely fresher than the air inside.

Planning for Health

The plan of a house describes the organization of spaces within the house, their shapes and the ways in which they connect. We have seen how zoning the site to build buffers between potential pollution sources and the house can minimize problems. The first principle to keep in mind while planning the healthy house is to zone the activities of the house from a health-oriented point of view. Some activities are more likely than others to generate or introduce outside contaminants into the living space. Just as a site can be zoned to buffer the house from environmental exposures, the house should be organized to separate "dirty" and "clean" activities.

The cleanest space in the house should most likely be the bedroom. This is the place where people usually spend the most time. For the extremely hypersensitive, and people with health problems that confine their movements, the bedroom becomes the primary therapeutic environment; the "sanctuary." In many cases, it is the only room that people can afford to completely detoxify, making it the most common renovation priority. For all of us, harried in our daily lives, the bedroom should be a final refuge of comfort and quiet. Consider it as though it were your only room: it might ideally have a window on the east to help you rise in the morning, and a window placed toward the cleanest and quietest orientation, so that fresh air carries you to sleep at night. The bedroom should probably be placed away from the activity of the social spaces and the heat and odors of the kitchen.

The sanctuary bedroom is often the simplest and least cluttered room of the house, providing the fewest possible extraneous materials to offgas and surfaces to collect dust. Closet spaces in many healthy houses are removed from the bedroom proper, isolating the room from potential odors carried in on clothing, or mustiness generated in untended corners. In the Barrhaven Apartments (Case Study 3), for example, the closet opens to the hall

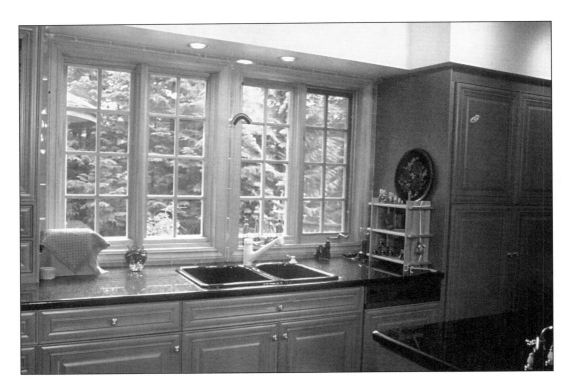

The healthy kitchen provides generous daylight and view, and is made with low toxicity, easily maintained materials. Morning sun is often desirable in the kitchen.

adjacent to the bedroom, and fresh air is drawn first through the bedroom, then into the closet and exhausted. When the closet is located in the bedroom, it is often fitted with an exhaust fan or duct to the ventilator to keep air moving away from the bedroom.

Besides closets, other potentially contaminating spaces include garages, entry areas, storage areas, kitchens, baths, laundry rooms, hobby areas, and home office areas housing pollutant-generating equipment such as copy machines and laser printers. In conventional housing these spaces tend to be poorly ventilated and filled with indoor air contaminants.

Garages are clearly a threat to indoor air quality, as an automobile will offgas a whole range of fumes, especially while it cools down after use. Garages should be physically distant from the house, or be separated from it with a well-constructed air barrier wall, and be well ventilated to the outside. The upscale suburban ideal of a three-car garage with the master bedroom above is asking for trouble. If you already have this situation, great care must be taken to ensure that there are no paths for air to travel upward through the construction.

An entry area, generous enough to comfortably remove and store coats and shoes, minimizes the dirt and outside odors brought into the house, and serves energy efficiency goals in colder climates. Kitchens, baths and laundries are sources of large amounts of moisture (see Ventilation in chapter 8 for how to deal with moisture), and are repositories of numerous cleaning and maintenance products that should be reviewed for their toxicity and added scents. Remember that the house is ultimately only as healthy as the things that you store in it.

Once the rooms are arranged, from dirty to clean, their degree of separation and connection should be carefully designed. Healthy houses generally have two distinct strategies, in recognition that there are two different basic concerns about the relation between the plan and the movement of air. On one hand, there are contaminants that clearly need to be isolated and contained. On the other hand, isolated, contained spaces which are poorly ventilated can themselves be a source of poor air quality.

One strategy is to create as much physical separation as possible between different rooms and their activities. In warm climates, where the cost of heating is not a concern, this can lead to breaking the house into a series of discreet pavilions. This is the logic of any house with a separate structure used as a home office, or painting studio, or any house with a detached garage/workshop. In a cold climate, separation might be achieved internally through the use of walls and tight-fitting doors to define each room. Doors isolating the kitchen and its cooking odors from the rest of the house can be particularly important and are often overlooked. Of course the heating and ventilating system must be equally separated for these isolated areas to operate independently.

The opposite strategy is to create as open and lofty a space as possible in order to promote air circulation and prevent mustiness. This is a strategy that is most effective in a warm climate, where all of the living spaces flow together, and all can be opened to outdoor patios and decks.

Providing adequate space for activities that support keeping the house clean is also essential. Clean air mechanical equipment such as air filters and central vacuum systems require some additional space, though not a great deal. Glass-enclosed display cases are an old fashioned example of storage that controls dust accumulation. At Barrhaven (Case Study 3), the display case is connected to the exhaust ventilation system so that the television, which produces "fried dust," can remain in the house.

Many people find it important to have a space where new belongings can be aired out before they are brought into the house. At Ecology House in San Rafael, California (Case Study 9) an open-air storage room is provided for the tenants for this purpose. At the Pitman House (Case Study 8), most of the family's personal belongings were initially stored in a separate outbuilding so the family could make the transition to the new house without having to discard their collected belongings. A storage loft can also play an ongoing role in keeping the house uncluttered and family memories intact.

The most successful healthy houses make provisions for members of the family who have needs and activities that may be in conflict with the goals of indoor air quality. This might lead to a detached home office or specially zoned and ventilated hobby room. For one couple it means a place where the spouse who travels, and is constantly subjected to cigarette smoke, can disrobe and bathe before entering the core of the house. For a retired couple, one of whom is extremely ill, it means two small houses, side by side, that allow both to enjoy cooking in their own way. These simple physical accommodations of personal differences can help to support special health needs and strong relationships.

Consider the idea of a healthy house that will suit a variety of generations, and allow you to age gracefully. This introduces the topic of "universal design," which is concerned with designing for differences in physical ability. Examples of accommodation are different heights of work surfaces, and easily managed door handles and water taps. These items can be retrofitted relatively easily as the need arises. However, the principles are worth considering as you design your house, even if you are not presently concerned with losing your mobility. Universal design suggests spaces that are large enough and open enough for easy movement. Kitchens and baths are larger than minimum, and have features such as walk-in showers that accommodate wheelchair access. Passages are wider, rooms tend to be directly connected so that movement is not difficult, and master bedrooms and/or water closets might be located on the ground floor. Living rooms might also be designed in such a way that they can be converted to bedrooms at a later date. Or provisions for small residential elevators can be built in, and occupied temporarily by closets if the elevator is not yet needed. Thresholds between spaces are made flush, a feature meant for wheelchairs, but enjoyed by anyone who has stumbled while walking through a doorway.

Consider providing for a separate apartment or an anticipated extension as a part of the house plan. The so-called "granny flat" has returned to the housing market, recognizing that for various economic and social reasons, extended families are often returning to closer living arrangements. Alternately, if part of the house that is required by the size of the household now can be easily separated and rented out when the household has shrunk, it may make it financially easier to remain in the house. You may not want or be able to afford an extended house now, but planning for it can make it easier to accomplish later.

The bedroom should be thought of as a "sanctuary" from activity, noise and air pollution, especially for the hypersensitive.

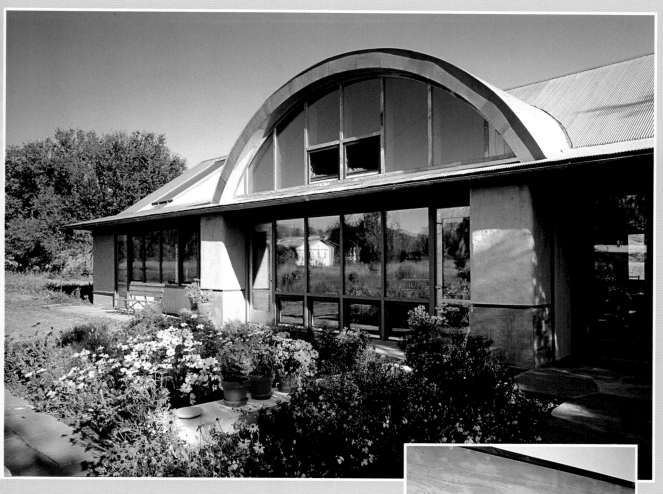

The principles involved in creating healthy, energy conserving and resource efficient houses are just abstractions until you actually face the challenge of creating a home. Building a healthy home entails a collision of needs: for human health, environmental and climactic considerations, and financial constraints. The process of harmonizing these demands makes design interesting and healthy houses showcases for innovative problem-solving. Some stunning examples are obviously expensive; others are elegantly economical. Some houses celebrate the freedom of living outside in balmy climates; others cheer winter spirits with their inner warmth. Some houses flaunt convention and express their owners' flair and daring; others choose to blend in, preferring the comfort of tradition. When you look at what can actually be done, it is clear that the challenges inherent in creating healthy houses do not limit design, but inspire it.

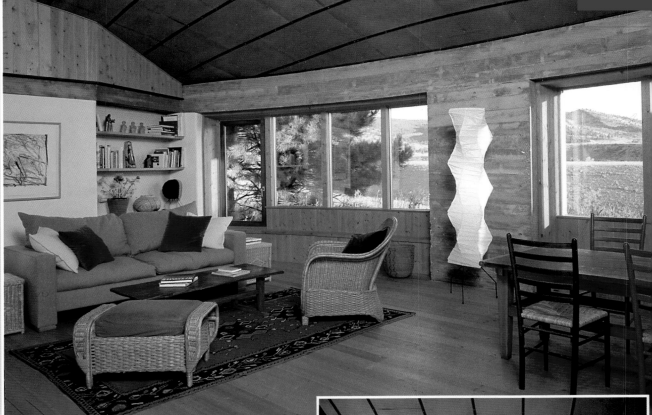

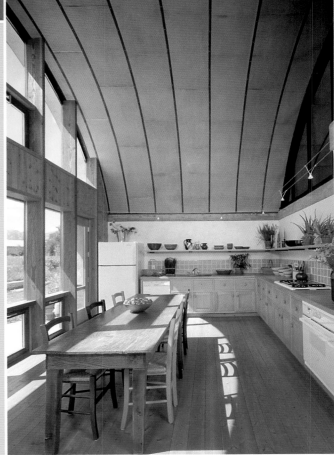

Jim Logan and Sherry Wiggins, an architect and a sculptor respectively, designed their home outside Boulder, Colorado to be healthy, energy efficient and gentle on the land. (See photos on previous page also.)

All the materials and finishes in the house are non-toxic and natural, and require little maintenance. The interior walls are finished with unpainted plaster colored with local river sand. The natural woodwork throughout is stained with plant and mineral pigments, and finished with linseed oil. The wood is solid and exposed to view. The few color accents on the walls and ceilings of the house are made with traditional milk-based paints.

The exterior walls are thick double adobe bricks, separated by a cavity insulated with chopped cellulose. Interior partitions are rammed earth. The massive walls, east/west elongation of the plan and high-performance insulated glazing create a textbook example of a passively heated solar house. Finally, the house is resource conserving in its use of locally available renewable materials.

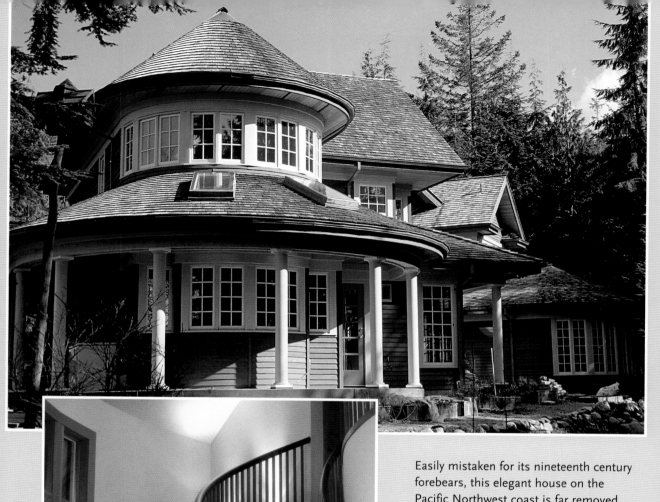

Easily mistaken for its nineteenth century forebears, this elegant house on the Pacific Northwest coast is far removed from the unconventional look and feel of the Logan/Wiggins house (opposite). It is, in fact, even more rigorously healthy, as it has been built to offer a safe haven for someone with extreme chemical sensitivities.

Though lush, the Pacific Northwest can be gray and gloomy for much of the year. This house is light-filled and cheery. It is also designed to carefully separate clean activities from irritant-producing activities, to be inherently non-toxic and easily cleaned and to offer complete control over the indoor environment for the occupants while maintaining energy efficiency standards. See Case Study 1 for an in-depth description of this house.

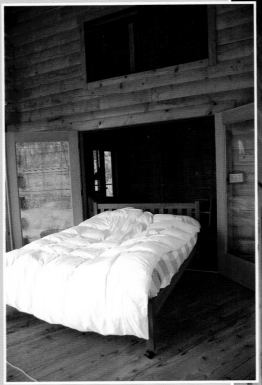

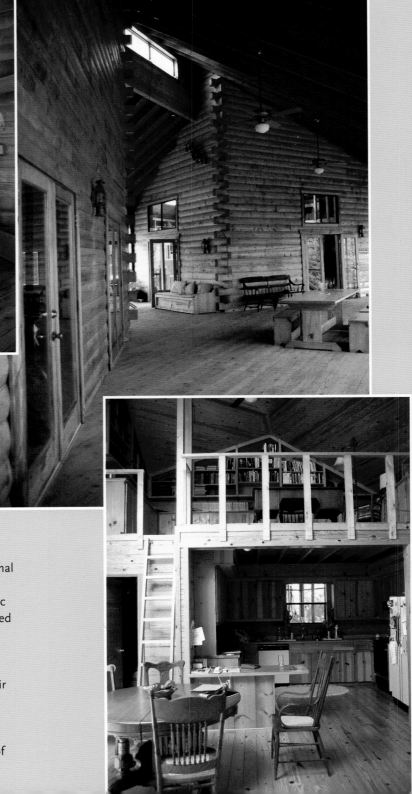

The Pitman Residence is a unique response to the hot and humid climate of the Hill Country of Texas. It uses the local vernacular to produce a strikingly contemporary house. Here, the climate and the owner's sense of design come together to create a house ideally suited to a family seeking refuge from ailments caused by exposure to pesticides and other chemicals.

The house is composed of two traditional log cabins raised high off the ground to catch summer breezes and aid in non-toxic pest control efforts. The cabins are gathered under a single roof, and surrounded by a screened porch that serves as the primary living space of the house. This outdoor room makes the most of the site's fresh air and mild climate, allowing year-round outdoor living. The construction of the house uses only non-toxic materials. See Case Study 8 for an in-depth description of this house.

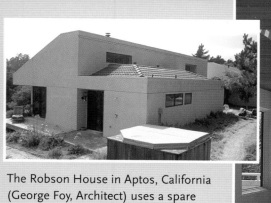

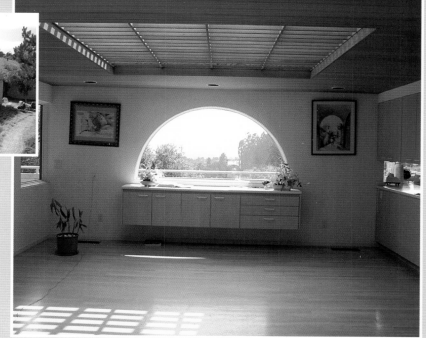

The Robson House in Aptos, California (George Foy, Architect) uses a spare modernist design to create an open-plan house. This openness serves health-related needs of a chemically sensitive client. The house is naturally well ventilated and easily cleaned. In addition, the house incorporates wheelchair accessibility without compromising the elegance of the design.

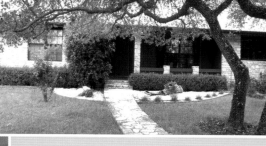

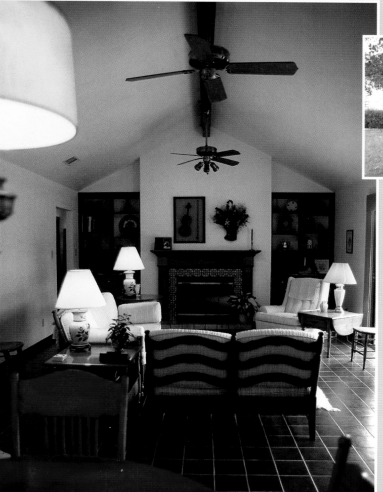

Located in the Texas Hill Country, the Oetzel house proves that the highest standards of health can be achieved on a reasonable budget in a house that is perfectly at home in its neighborhood. The guiding philosophy is that care in selecting materials and construction is the key to health.

Much like the Pitman house (opposite page), this house promotes pesticide-free outdoor living and energy efficient sensitivity to the local climate. The house achieves a subtle beauty using non-toxic and easily maintained hard finishes such as unpainted plaster and ceramic tile. See Case Study 7 for an in-depth description of this house.

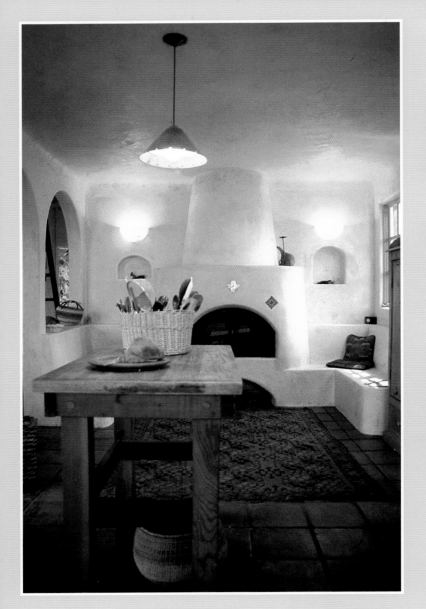

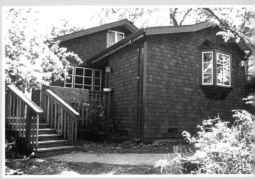

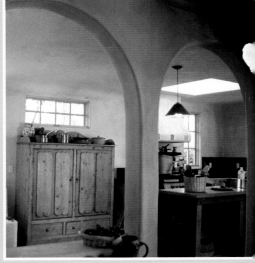

Renovation work presents its own unique set of challenges for healthy housing. This Sonoma County remodel preserves the time-honored warmth of an existing house while fixing potential health problems and inventing a new sense of space within.

Saving old structures may be resource efficient but it is often difficult to make such buildings healthy and energy efficient. Health is addressed here by fixing major moisture-related problems, and the dark, awkward kitchen is recreated as a light and airy family hearth. This newly spacious room features the varying textures and colors of hand-crafted forms and natural finishes. See Case Study 5 for an in-depth description of this house.

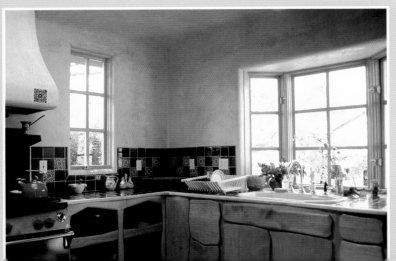

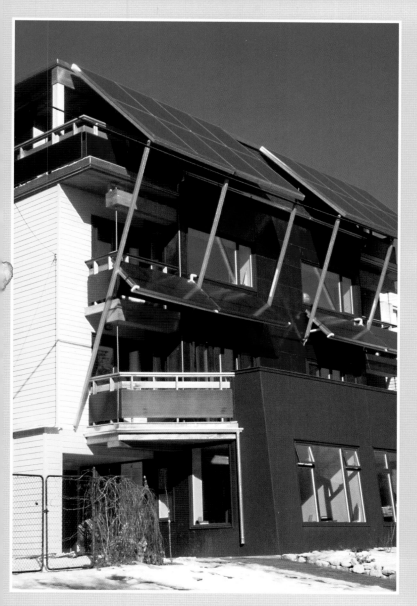

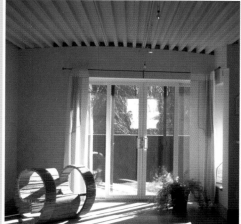

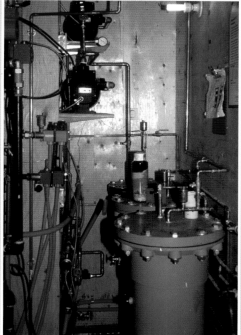

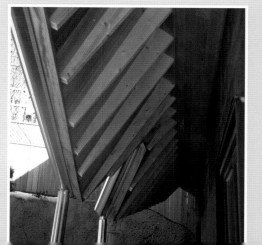

The Toronto Healthy House pushes state-of-the-art resource and energy efficiency to new heights while remaining faithful to the goals of healthy house construction. As a demonstration project, this passively heated duplex in the frigid climate of Toronto is both expensive and aesthetically bold.

Built on an 'unbuildable' urban infill lot, the hidden environmental costs of new development are eliminated. More radically, the two dwellings are completely self sufficient, generating their own electricity, capturing rain and snow melt for domestic use and recycling all waste water. At the same time, they use materials and finishes that are non-toxic, easily cleaned and naturally pest resistant. See Case Study 6 for an in-depth description of this house.

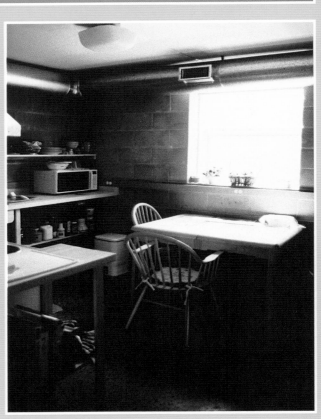

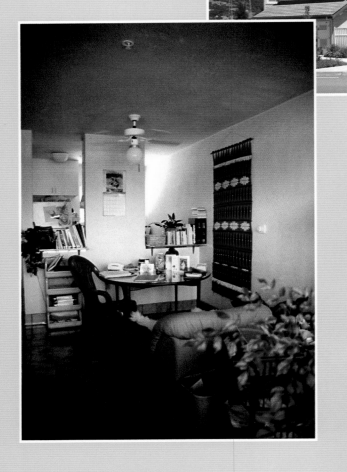

These two groundbreaking apartment buildings (one in the extremely cold climate of Ottawa, Ontario and the other in the mild climate of the San Francisco Bay area) demonstrate the potential for healthy housing to serve the needs of those debilitated by environmental hypersensitivities who don't have the money to create private sanctuaries. Both projects provide low-income housing for people with multiple chemical sensitivities. Both were constructed on strict budgets, and both respond to the specifics of climate. These constraints have created two buildings with different aesthetic expressions.

The features that unite Barrhaven (bottom) and Ecology House (top) are central themes in healthy housing. Both demonstrate great care in site selection, thoughtful control and use of the local climate, intelligent planning to separate potential contaminants from the living spaces, hard, non-toxic, easily cleaned surfaces and carefully conceived mechanical systems. Both face the unique challenge of designing for the unknown sensitivities of future residents, rather than the specific requirements of a single client. See Case Study 3 (Barrhaven) and Case Study 9 (Ecology House) for an in-depth description of each project.

Case Studies

CASE STUDY 1
New Detached Home

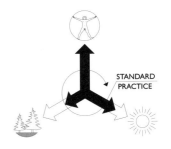

STANDARD PRACTICE

Name: single family, detached home

Location: Pacific Northwest coast

Seneca and Richard are a professional couple with a strong interest in health. Seneca was diagnosed with multiple chemical sensitivities in 1988 after she and Richard had moved into their dream home in a new subdivision. Her health had been deteriorating and it became worse in the new house, which had been designed with no special health emphasis. The couple was forced to move into rental accommodation in another part of the city, and they eventually sold their dream home. As a temporary measure, they converted a small outbuilding into a clean-air safe room for Seneca in which she lived for eight years. During this time, she began specialized treatments and began slowly to recover. Seneca and Richard knew that their next home would have to be designed specifically for health.

DESIGN PROCESS

Seneca and Richard were involved in the site selection, design and construction of their home. They familiarized themselves with the special housing needs of the chemically sensitive, and Richard took home-building courses so he could better instruct the architect and work with the builder. He studied building science and energy efficiency, as well as heating and ventilation.

The goal was to build a home that would give Seneca control over her entire environment, rather than just a few safe rooms she would be confined to. Seneca and Richard chose a healthy-building consultant and architect, and began to look for a site. Their eventual choice was a one-acre lot in a semi-rural location on the edge of a major city. The area is quiet and has good air quality, except for occasional wood smoke from the neighbors.

Light and color were also major design considerations. In fall, winter and spring, the Pacific Northwest coast has a cloudy climate with limited periods of sunshine. Based on research and personal experience, Seneca knew that a home with maximum natural light would be beneficial to her, mentally and physically. This, combined with carefully selected, cheerful

Design Team:
 Graeme Bristol, Architect; Marnie Tamaki, David Rousseau
Builder: Helmut Schein, Helma Construction

70

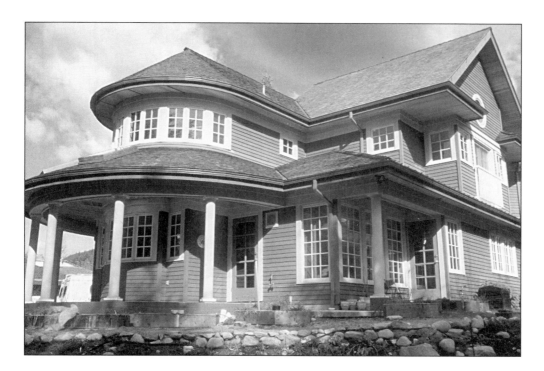

colors has resulted in a peaceful, healing atmosphere. The generous use of windows also brings the surrounding forest into the home, further enhancing this atmosphere.

Another major design concept in the house is "plan zoning" or separating the spaces from one another to maintain air quality. The two wings contain separate rooms for an art studio and sun room. Rooms that contain potential irritants are highly separated from rooms that don't, such as the bedroom. The kitchen and entry hall are at the center of the house. Areas that accommodate such activities as cooking, laundry and working at the computer, which might affect Seneca due to air pollution and noise, are all separately exhausted. The heating and air systems are zoned for each room and do not recirculate air.

The home is crescent shaped, and opens to the south for solar access. It is only one room deep in most areas to take maximum advantage of available daylight and sunlight. This placement also allows for good cross-ventilation when weather permits. The covered porches shelter rooms from rain, but have skylights to let light in. Most rooms open out onto porches, terraces or balconies because the climate is benign and relatively insect free. The bright exterior color scheme contrasts with the dark conifer trees and gray skies.

The home is built on an insulated, heated slab, with no basement or crawl space, to minimize the risk of drainage problems and fungus. It is

South view, entering the courtyard. This home makes maximum use of sunlight and daylight in a cloudy climate.

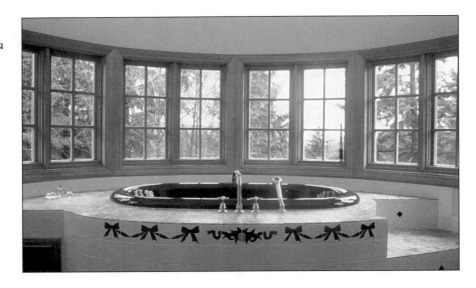

finished with ceramics, stone and hardwoods to minimize emissions and maintenance, and has an isolated boiler room for the heating and vacuuming equipment. The garage, with its workshop and garden storage, is fully separated.

Seneca spent many hours sitting in her garden with the architect and a sketch book to develop the design. The initial concepts were fairly conventional, with the healthy building technology added on. Slowly, as each scheme was developed and sketched for review, more conventional house forms were abandoned and the unique crescent form and conical roofs evolved. When Seneca and Richard were satisfied with the basic concept, the builder and other consultants began working on all of the required features, coordinated by the architect. Preliminary costing was done at the beginning of the design development, and accurate costing after most of the details had been decided. A set of healthy building specifications were prepared, with special instructions, as part of the construction contract.

MATERIALS SELECTION

Material selection was done based on Seneca's experience with her temporary home and by research. Seneca challenge tested any materials she thought she might be sensitive to (see chapter 9). Most conventional paints were rejected, but solid hardwoods and softwoods with safe finishes were acceptable. Most interior caulkings were rejected and had to be replaced with acceptable sealant tape. Flexible rubber tubing for carrying heating water through the framing was also rejected in favor of copper pipe.

MECHANICAL SYSTEMS

Seneca and Richard do not like appliance noise and the home needed to be highly zoned to prevent odors and noise from migrating between rooms. To address these needs, a hot water heating system was chosen which provides zone-controlled heat to the concrete slabs, baseboard convectors upstairs, domestic hot water, and low-temperature sauna heat, all from one boiler. There are two oversized ventilation systems, one for each wing. They supply outdoor air to each room, after passing it through seven filters, and exhaust air (with heat recovery) to the outside from the laundry, bathrooms, storage closets and kitchen. The kitchen has a high-capacity commercial kitchen exhaust, and the sun room and exercise rooms have thermostatic, reversible cooling fans. There is a laboratory-style fume hood in the art studio to allow Seneca to handle selected drawing inks and ceramic glazes.

There is a whole house water filter, and a three-stage kitchen filter for drinking water. A central vacuum is located in the furnace room and is ducted to the outside.

CONSTRUCTION AND SUPERVISION

The contractor was chosen for his experience with energy efficient construction, and because he built Seneca's special sanctuary room at their previous home. He is an exacting project manager who is extremely attentive to details, and he has long-term relationships with his sub-trades. The construction contract was not put to open bidding. The contractor provided a detailed "fixed price" quote for the house to "lockup stage": and then a "cost plus" fee arrangement for all subsequent finishing work, much of which was controlled by Seneca and Richard (see chapter 10).

The general contractor was on the site daily, and brought any significant questions directly back to the design team. There was no smoking on site, or use and storage of hazardous materials. The trades were all instructed by the general contractor about the special nature of the project, and encouraged to ask questions and make suggestions.

In general, the project went very well, due to careful preparation and exacting management. The contractor had some difficulty with special materials and procedures, such as the low-toxicity sealer for the plywood which could not be sprayed. It was finally brushed and rolled onto all necessary surfaces. Special paints were imported which also required special handling. Small amounts were tinted on-site for special uses such as colored walls in the dining room and office. The oil and beeswax finish used on some of the hardwood floors seemed acceptable when tested, but produced odor problems when applied to a large area which took several months of airing out to finally resolve. During this time Seneca could not use one of the bedrooms. It was determined that the problem was probably a natural aromatic oil in the finish.

The major construction problem was that some finishing decisions, such as decorative tiles and hardwood stair design, were postponed, and then proved difficult to resolve. This delayed other finishing steps. Also, the cabinets were built to special specifications and delivery was delayed. The special low-toxicity sauna and some other items were not chosen until construction was nearly complete, and these delays required the contractor and trades to return more often than would otherwise have been necessary.

Due to the special healthy features, this project cost approximately 12% more to build than a comparable, custom home with high-quality finishes.

STAR DIAGRAM ASSESSMENT AND CRITIQUE

The owners are delighted with the home, and feel that Seneca finally has the control over her home environment which she needs. The main air quality problem has been periodic wood smoke from neighbors in the area which gets inside the house. A recirculating furnace system could have provided more successful filtration when the house is closed up than the prefilters on the intake air system are able to do, but this would have compromised the zoning and isolation design. There have been several small technical problems to resolve, such as chronic mildew on the exterior porch columns (which were finished with a low-toxicity exterior stain), and several breakdowns and noise problems with the heating system.

THE SUMMARY TABLE

Project

New detached home, one occupant with multiple chemical sensitivities.

Climate and Site

Pacific Northwest rain forest, approx. 55 in. (1400 mm) annual precipitation, 20°F (−7°C) winter low, 80°F (26°C) summer high. One-acre treed lot in a semi-rural area, distant from highways, industry and agriculture. South slope with adequate drainage, minimal termite problems.

The Building

New construction, 1994. 2800 sq.ft. (260 sq.m.), two bedrooms, two baths, laundry, kitchen, dining room, sun room, art studio, living room, library, pantry, exercise room, low-temperature sauna and isolated utility room. Detached two-car garage with shop and garden storage.

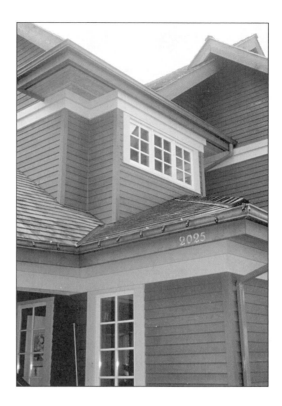

Design Emphasis

Climatic Design— maximizes solar exposure, daylight, cross-ventilation and rain shelter.

Energy Efficient Design—insulation and draft sealing are to high-efficiency standards (computer modeling was done). Gas boiler is 94% efficient.

Resource Efficient Design—little effort was made to use resource efficient materials or include water conservation techniques and systems.

North view, facing the road. Bold and complex roof lines match the strong color scheme chosen for this home.

Air Quality Design—rigorous space planning, materials testing and heating, ventilation and filtration design to reduce maintenance and indoor pollution.

Design for Isolation of Pollutants—highly separated plan, exhaust from all storage spaces, studio, exercise room and sunroom and bathrooms. Some "encapsulated" materials, e.g. sealed plywood subfloors.

Design for Light—shallow rooms, large glass areas, clear glass.

Design for Noise Protection—no special effort required.

Design for EMF Protection—no special effort required.

Design for Low Maintenance—ceramic and stone floors, built-in vacuum.

Other Design Emphasis—bright and contrasting colors.

Materials Selection

Foundations—concrete slab without additives, mineral oil concrete form release, heavy-duty ground moisture barrier.

Frame—2x6 wood walls, 2x10 and 2x12 floor and roof joists, roof trusses, plywood sheathing and subfloors sealed with low-toxicity sealer.

Roofing—wood shingles, copper flashings.

Exterior Finishes—cedar siding and soffitts, latex stain.

Insulation—polystyrene slab, polyolefin weather barrier, fiberglass batts, airtight drywall with taped polyethylene air/vapor barrier.

Windows and Doors—solid wood and new custom-built wood sash window, double glazed, solid wood and metal entrance and interior doors.

Interior Finishes—gypsum board with low-toxicity sealer and paints for ceilings and walls, zero VOCs paint, all-natural paint and tint, hardwood and softwood trims, all-natural sealer.

Floor Coverings—ceramic tile and slate in thinset mortar main floor, cement and sand grout, hardwood second floor, all natural sealer and beeswax, no carpet.

Cabinets—hardwood, formaldehyde-free fiberboard, granite tops, low-toxicity finishes.

Furnishings—antique solid wood furniture, safe finishes and glues, rattan with organic cotton futon cushions and metal frame furniture. Custom hardwood futon bed.

Other—low-temperature sauna with heated tile floor, hardwood benches, fiber cement board sheathing with hardwood paneling, custom hardwood futon bed and polyester fiber insulation.

Heating, Air Conditioning, Air Filtration and Ventilation

Heating, A/C Type—condensing gas boiler in isolated furnace room, stainless domestic hot water tank and exchanger, in-floor radiant slab (polybutylene tubing), perimeter convectors (copper tubing).

Ventilation System Type—two heat exchange ventilators ducted to all rooms, exhausts in kitchen, laundry, closets and utility room. Supplies in bedrooms, living room, library, dining room, independent exhaust fans in kitchen, sunroom, exercise room and art studio.

Filtration System Type—seven-stage fabric and carbon pre-filters in ventilator supply. High-quality portable air filters.

Other Mechanical Notes—built-in vacuum in isolated room with outside exhaust. Whole house water filter and kitchen filter.

CASE STUDY 2
Vancouver Healthy House

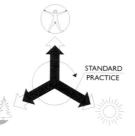

STANDARD
PRACTICE

Name: Vancouver Healthy House
Demonstration Project, new home

Location: Vancouver, BC, Canada, coastal temperature

The Vancouver Healthy House is a demonstration project illustrating intensive urban land use, resource efficiency, energy efficiency and healthy building features. The project was built by a private developer and was partially funded by The Canada Mortgage and Housing Corporation (CMHC), Canada's national housing research demonstration agency. It was used for teaching and research and has now been sold. The design was one of the two winners of the 1992 CMHC Healthy Housing Competition emphasizing "healthy planet, healthy city and healthy people."

All of the design features, construction methods, systems and materials used were closely scrutinized for energy, resource, and water efficiency, CO_2 release and solid waste production. The design had to be reasonably simple, currently feasible, and accessible to any homeowner and builder—no extraordinary approaches or prototype components were used. The house is an "urban infill"; it is placed on a rear yard behind an existing 1920s house. The infill aspect demonstrates efficient land use, heritage preservation, and presents cash-poor homeowners with an income opportunity through rental or subdivision and sale. The original house was also renovated as part of the project, with the goal of making both houses combined use less energy and water than the original house alone had. The heating and ventilating systems, low-toxicity materials and whole house water treatment system meet high standards for health and comfort, though they were not specifically designed for the environmentally hypersensitive.

DESIGN PROCESS

The design team prepared a design for the competition using a typical site, though no zoning approval or developer had been secured. After they won the CMHC competition, the design team searched for an investor with a property located where the city would allow a coach-house-type infill unit. An investor was found and negotiations began with the planning depart-

Design Team:
   Greg Johnson,
   Architect;
   Christopher
   Mattock, David
   Rousseau
Builder: Warren Jones,
   Cortez Energy
   Efficient Homes
CMHC Project
   Managers: James
   Robar, Christopher
   Ives
Technical
   Assistance and
   Communications:
   Canada Mortgage
   and Housing
   Corporation

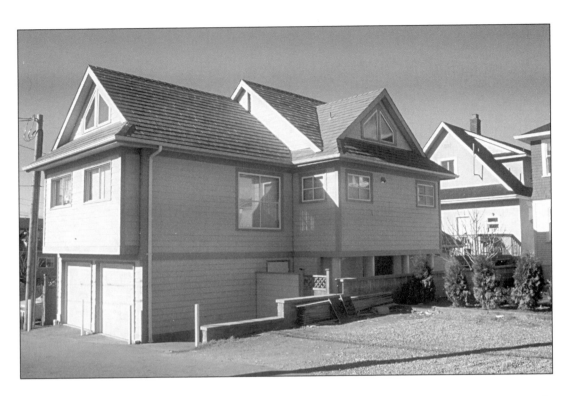

Southeast view showing existing 1920s house on the right.

ment. The size, placement, height and roofline of the house were precisely defined by the agreement struck with the city using local design guidelines. Negotiations with the fire department were much more difficult, because the new house does not face a principal street. The fire department was not confident that the house would be accessible by emergency vehicles, even though it faces two 20-foot-wide lanes. Eventually, a compromise was reached by providing a fire-protected sideyard next to the main house to allow firefighters to reach the unit from the main street.

Once the planning and fire access problems were solved, the design team began by placing the windows and solar domestic water preheater for optimal exposure. Solar planning and the entire energy efficient design were done using computer modeling. The final floor plan has one bedroom, a laundry, and a bath on the main level, and a loft, which could be a bedroom/sitting room, an office or a playroom. The height and size of the loft was limited by the building height restrictions and the maximum floor area allowed under the zoning regulations.

An open web floor and roof framing system was chosen, because it uses less wood than solid joists and it allows pipes and ducts to pass easily through the floors without requiring dropped ceilings. A fully integrated heating and ventilation system was chosen using a solar collector to preheat hot water. The design called for high-performance windows, and siding and roofing made of extremely durable fiber-cement. The exterior walls are braced with steel brackets and have little plywood sheathing; instead they have exterior insulating board. The wall system also uses advanced framing (optimum value engineering) methods to conserve wood, combined with an "airtight drywall" system for climate control and to reduce air leaks, and a "rain screen" system to minimize weather damage. The insulation in the walls and roof is a fiberized cellulose, blown-in system, and the slab is insulated with ozone-safe polystyrene board.

MATERIALS SELECTION

The exterior and structural materials were chosen for their durability, and resource efficiency. The interior materials were chosen for their low-maintenance requirements and minimal indoor pollution. The materials are not as rigorously healthy as a hypersensitive person might require, but were chosen with prevention in mind. For example, a natural linoleum was used in some areas because it is very durable and made from renewable materials. However, it does have a mild linseed oil odor which lingers for several weeks which is unacceptable for some sensitive people, so it was aged and sealed to reduce the problem. Some conventional gypsum board was also used, which may not be acceptable to a sensitive person, but it was sealed with a low-toxicity acrylic sealer to reduce odor and control moisture absorption.

MECHANICAL SYSTEMS

A fan-coil heating system was chosen with a hot water loop because it does not cook dust, and it provides filtration of recirculated air. This is important in an urban location, because outdoor air quality is often poor. A heat recovery ventilator provides outdoor air to the fan-coil, and exhausts the bathroom, laundry and kitchen. A single, sealed combustion boiler provides both space heat and water heating, and is connected to a solar preheater tank. The fan-coil contains an effective bag filter for dust and a carbon filter for odors. The combined heating and domestic hot water system was new to the plumbing inspectors and had to be verified by the designers. It is fitted with a pump timer which operates the coil briefly once per day, even when no heat is required, to prevent stagnation of the water in the coil. The plumbing had to be modified slightly after installation to prevent unintentional heating in summer when a flow was induced by using domestic hot

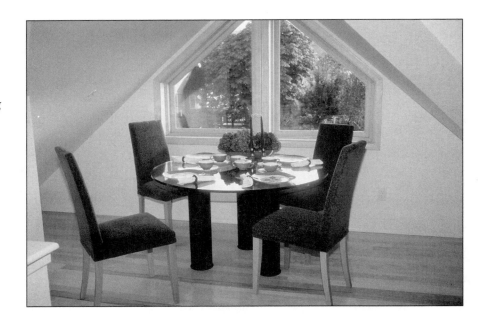

water. These systems are now available as a factory-made package, including all components and controls.

CONSTRUCTION AND SUPERVISION

The builder was chosen for his extensive experience with energy efficient construction and his ability to adopt innovative practices when needed. He selected and instructed the tradespeople carefully, and supervised closely during construction. The advanced framing systems presented some difficulties because several of the details had to be worked out on the job site. The frame was also unusually flexible (though never unsafe) until the cladding and roof strapping were all in place, causing some worry among the carpenters. It required experimentation to master the cutting and fastening of the fiber cement products, and the blown insulation required a special high-powered blower and forced settling technique. These factors necessitated flexibility and ingenuity on the part of the builder, added to cost and slowed construction somewhat.

Many of the unusual materials were donated, or partly donated by manufacturers, which required a lot of communication and coordination. Some were shipped long distances, which was considered an acceptable compromise in order to showcase things not made locally, but which are locally appropriate.

The complex roof design with vaulted ceilings and the two-car garage be-

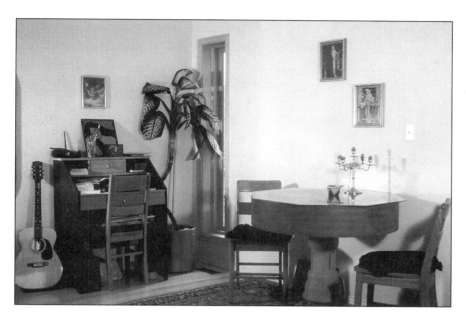

The owners use simple, traditional furnishings in uncluttered settings in this compact home.

low resulted in several structural problems. These were solved with a few heavy laminated beams. The beams were used as ridge and valley timbers, to support floors and to transfer loads to bearing walls. A large truss using steel rod ties was used to support the main roof. These structural solutions used more lumber and steel than would have been required for a less complex design. The compromise was considered acceptable to meet city requirements and the desired spatial qualities and character of the house.

The construction cost, including the value of donations, was approximately 21% above a typical construction of similar quality without all of the unusual features.

STAR DIAGRAM ASSESSMENT AND CRITIQUE

Judging from discussion during the public open houses and the professional tours, the project was a success. Visitors remarked that they were impressed with the range of healthy features demonstrated by the house, including intensive land use, energy and resource efficiency, innovative materials and construction methods, and indoor air quality. Many commented on the successful design features of the house and the spacious and bright feeling. A frequent observation was "it smells fresh, not like a new house." Criticisms were raised over the noisy and congested location and the small back yard remaining between the existing house and the infill unit.

The painters commented on the excellent coverage and sealing properties as well as the safe and easy handling of the low-toxicity paints. Since completion, the indoor air has been measured and monitored and contained less than 40% of the typical volatile air pollution found in new housing after three months. Dust levels are extremely low and it is a very quiet house, especially given the amount of traffic surrounding the site. The water usage and energy performance have also been monitored and are very good, except for some spring and fall overheating problems due to limited solar shading and limited use by occupants of the operable windows for venting due to noise and pollution at the site.

THE SUMMARY TABLE

For Whom?

A healthy house for demonstration and eventual sale.

Climate and Site

The climate is Pacific Northwest rain forest, approximately 55 inches (1400 mm) annual precipitation, 20°F (–7°C) winter low, 80°F (26°C) summer high. A 3800-square-foot lot in an urban area close to major streets and commercial lanes. Southern exposure.

The Building

1500 square feet (140 sq.m.), one bedroom and loft bedroom/office, living room, kitchen, laundry, two baths and storage room. Attached two-car garage with utility room.

Design Emphasis

Climatic Design—passive solar design, rain screen protection, enclosed balcony, daylight design, highly insulated.

Energy Efficient Design—superinsulated, high-performance windows, solar water heater, highly efficient boiler.

Resource Efficient Design—reduced wood use, use of recycled content and highly durable materials, water conserving fixtures.

Air Quality Design—low-toxicity materials and finishes, low-temperature heat, fully ducted ventilation system, filtration, recirculation system with high-performance dust and carbon odor removal filters, glass cooktop electric stove.

Design for Isolation of Pollutants—extremely draft-sealed envelope to control infiltration of polluted air.

Design for Light—large windows, shallow rooms, light colored surfaces.

Design for Noise Protection—noise-resistant windows and doors, exterior insulation to reduce sound through walls, sound-absorbing gypsum underlay between floors.

Design for Low Maintenance—minimal carpeting, sealed, low-porosity surfaces.

Materials Selection

Foundations—concrete slab foundations with no additives.

Frame—advanced wood framing, open web joists, steel bracing system.

Roofing—fiber cement shingles.

Exterior Finishes—fiber cement plank siding with low-toxicity stain.

Insulation—type II polystyrene under slab, blown-in cellulose in walls and ceilings with airtight drywall draft sealing method.

Windows and Doors—wood sash, sealed thermally broken double-glazing with argon gas fill.

Interior Finishes—fiber gypsum board walls and ceilings, low-toxicity, vapor resistant sealer, zero VOCs paints, and all-natural millwork sealers.

Floor Coverings—sealed and aged natural linoleum in entry, kitchen, laundry and washrooms, natural wool carpet, prefinished birch veneer planks for upper floors.

Cabinets— formaldehyde-free fiber board, maple veneer fiber board, solid maple trims and frames, low-toxicity coatings

Heating, Air Conditioning, Air Filtration and Ventilation

Heating, A/C Type—fan-coil furnace with single boiler supplying both heat and hot water in a combined system. Sealed combustion, 94% efficient boiler, solar water preheater.

Ventilation System Type—heat exchange ventilator ducted to fan coil furnace.

Filtration System Type—85% efficient bag filters and carbon treated fabric.

C A S E   S T U D Y   3
Multi-Tenant Building

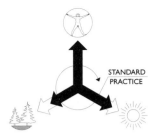

STANDARD
PRACTICE

Name: Barrhaven Community Housing
for the Environmentally Hypersensitive

Location: Nepean (in Ottawa/Carleton Region) Ontario, Canada,
cold climate

The Barrhaven Community Housing for the Environmentally Hypersensitive is part of a larger nonprofit special-needs housing development sponsored by the Barrhaven United Church congregation. Seven of the larger project's 41 units are housed in a unique building designed to accommodate those suffering from sensitivities to irritants such as dust, molds and chemical emissions. Built in the spirit of both social and environmental responsibility, the project allows people who might otherwise be institutionalized to live as part of the community, and serves as an experimental prototype for future moderate-cost healthy building projects.

DESIGN PROCESS

The architect had a keen interest in finding innovative and affordable solutions to design problems. The problem in this case was to plan for an undefined list of individual sensitivities without specific occupants to work with, and to do so under the tight financial constraints of a social housing project. A pioneering builder of healthy housing became involved with the design team after hearing the architect describe the challenge on a local talk radio program.

Since the future residents could not be consulted, the design team decided to take no chances by eliminating as many potential irritants as possible in the building. Their strategy was to build a simple structure and to use the savings to pay for exceptionally low-risk materials and healthy building construction practices. As many surfaces as possible were left in a natural, unfinished state. In addition, the designers sought to eliminate all of the hidden spaces where mold and mildew problems can go unchecked in conventional construction. This entailed eliminating basements and placing mechanical equipment inside each apartment. More radically, the resulting design eliminated all of the enclosed cavities within walls, under bathtubs

Design Team: Philip
Sharp, Architect;
Buchan, Lawton,
Parent Ltd.,
Consulting
Engineers
Builder: Drerup
Armstrong Limited

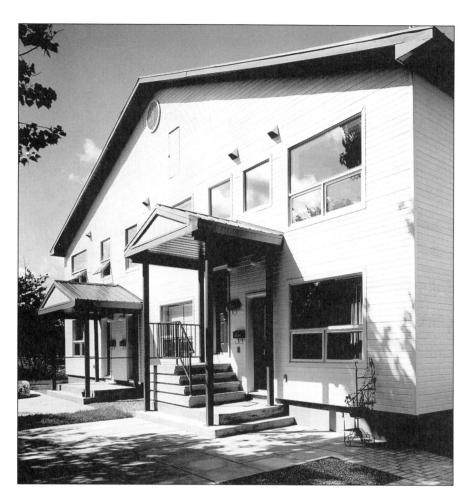

The Barrhaven apartments are two-story units with individual entries, allowing occupants greater control than in a building with common corridors.

and behind fixed appliances so that every inch of each apartment would be accessible for cleaning.

The resulting structure is a hard-surfaced box wrapped with a superinsulated shell, and equipped with mechanical ventilation that provides customizable filtration and heat recovery. The walls within the living spaces are either concrete masonry units with grouted solid cores or solid wood plank partitions such as you might find in a very old wooden house. Everything within the structure is exposed and to the greatest extent possible unfinished.

The basic unit is a rectangle plan with a consistent mechanical room layout that organizes all utilities, appliances, kitchens and bath fixtures. All of the appliances and fixtures protrude through the walls of either the mechanical room or other storage spaces, allowing complete access from behind for cleaning and maintenance. This core is the same for one-, two-, and three-bedroom units.

85

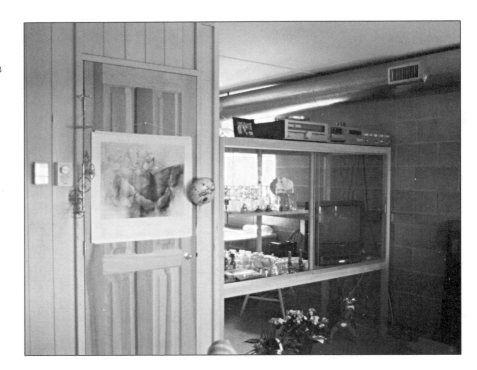

The vented television cabinet and an accessible refrigerator enclosure help make this a clean apartment.

The apartments each have a vestibule large enough for visitors to leave street clothes in which is served by a dedicated exhaust which isolates the dirt and moisture that would otherwise be tracked into the living space. At the opposite end of each dwelling the bedroom closet is treated as walk-in storage, opening onto the hall, leaving the bedroom as an isolated inner sanctuary.

MATERIALS SELECTION

Each of the materials were as additive free as possible. The concrete used for the first-floor slab, the precast second floor and in the concrete block walls contained none of the typical plasticizers or air-entraining agents. Organic soap was used in place of diesel fuel as a form release agent. The concrete floors were ground with a terrazzo grinder for an elegant and low-cost finish. Both the concrete walls and floors are sealed with a nontoxic sodium silicate solution.

A variety of nonresinous hardwoods were used, such as basswood for the plank walls and second-floor ceiling, poplar for doors, and the more expensive but more durable red maple for the stairs and kitchen counters. All of the woodwork relies on mechanical fasteners or white glue. Wood surfaces subject to wear were finished with water-based urethane and the remainder were sealed with the same sodium silicate solution as above.

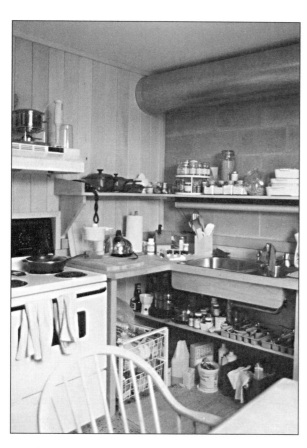

The kitchen area can be warm and personalized, while still incorporating healthy materials and systems.

The superinsulated envelope is made up of 2x8 wood framing filled with additive-free rock wool insulation. Where this is outside of the concrete block walls, a conventional polyethylene vapor barrier is used, and where it is exposed to the interior, foil-faced drywall is used as both vapor barrier and interior sheathing. The foil face of the drywall is installed to face the interior, isolating the entire assembly from the room to ensure that any conceivable offgassing is vented to the exterior.

There are only two painted surfaces inside the units. The steel structural frame that supports the floor at the stair opening was finished at an autobody shop with baked enamel. The underside of the concrete plank second floor was painted with zero VOCs acrylic paint, and it was painted only because the planks arrived at the job site unacceptably stained.

MECHANICAL SYSTEMS

Each dwelling has its own self-contained mechanical systems to avoid cross-contamination. These systems are central to the design of the project, completing the superinsulation strategy by providing both continuous fresh air to the living spaces and dedicated exhausts from areas where odors and moisture might accumulate.

The primary mechanical system is ducted forced-air heating, using a boiler and fan-coil furnace. The low-temperature heat exchange avoids most of the dust problems associated with conventional furnaces. The heated air is passed through a customizable filter bank and is then distributed.

The ventilation system consists of a heat recovery ventilator that exhausts air taken from the vestibule, storage areas, kitchen, laundry and bathroom. The kitchen is exhausted from behind the refrigerator in order to capture any odors from the drain pan. Exhaust is also provided for a built-in glass cabinet in the living room used to house televisions and other belongings prone to offgassing. This arrangement effectively ventilates all of the storage space of the house except the shelves under the kitchen counter, which are left open to promote air circulation.

Surprisingly, the range hood is not independently exhausted. Instead, a standard ductless carbon filter captures cooking fumes but otherwise relies on the general kitchen exhaust. Though less than ideal in theory, so far none of the residents has complained about excessive cooking odors as a source of irritation.

Air from all seven units is exhausted through a cupola that gathers together all of the roof penetrations for the buildings, while replacement air is drawn in through an intake in the gable-end wall. Exhaust lines for the dryer, and for the possible addition of a central vacuum system run in the slab and exit on the leeward side of the building, away from any operable windows.

The ductwork throughout the units is fully exposed and designed to be easily dismantled and cleaned by the occupant as often as desired.

CONSTRUCTION AND SUPERVISION

Careful management of the job site to prevent unintended contamination was critical at Barrhaven, where the most sensitive potential resident had to be provided for.

Key to the success of the project was the early involvement of the builder, the building inspector, local code officials and other consultants and advocacy groups that served as resources for the architect. The project would not have been feasible without Housing Ministry waivers that allowed the structure to be administered separately from the bulk of the project, and without open bids. It also allowed for performance-based specifications to be developed through the construction process, setting out the goals of the project but allowing a great deal of freedom in finding ways to satisfy them. These flexible arrangements enabled the architect and builder to solve problems collaboratively throughout the process of design and construction, and to involve subcontractors in the search for acceptable products and construction methods.

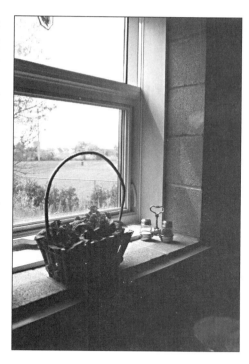

The builders employed a small crew that was fully aware of the healthy objectives of the project and enjoyed the level of craftsmanship required. Letters of commitment to objectives were similarly secured from each subcontractor. The architect describes the job site as rigorously clean. No cleaning fluids, lubricants or gasoline were allowed within the structure. All rest breaks were taken off site. Smoking was not allowed. Exhaust fumes from diesel delivery trucks and from the terrazzo grinder were ducted away from the site, and vehicles were not allowed to idle nearby. Tool and material storage was handled carefully, with all potentially problematic substances stored off site. A large container of soap was always on hand and people washed oil off their hands and tools constantly. Metal goods, such as the ductwork and roofing, were washed down before installation to remove machine oil residue, and the site superintendent even washed batches of drywall screws for the same reason.

Personal items are very carefully chosen by the environmentally hypersensitive.

One fluke accident on site illustrates the level of care taken. During the erection of the second-floor structure, a hose on the precast plank hoist burst, spraying hydraulic fluid into the air. Fortunately, the fluid sprayed away from the building, but a pallet of concrete blocks and several yards of topsoil were contaminated. They were removed and disposed of as a result. In addition to the thorough cleaning the site received, the already completed first floor slab was reground and polished as a precaution.

The architect later heard that the crew of the precast plant where the planks were made reportedly found it such an improvement to work without the permeating odor of diesel fuel that they continued the practice of using organic soap as a release agent after the order was filled. Unfortunately, the soap didn't protect the steel forms from rust, causing staining of the planks, which then had to be painted on site.

STAR DIAGRAM ASSESSMENT AND CRITIQUE

As a project reflecting a strong social and environmental commitment, Barrhaven scores highly in each point of the star diagram. It is designed to be as healthy as possible. The well-insulated building is extremely energy efficient. Its situation within a larger community and design for extreme economy helps to reduce the waste associated with its construction and use. The impact that this path-breaking project had is summed up by the outreach education done to persuade the neighbors and the local government not to use pesticides in the area during construction. This request led to a widespread and permanent move away from pesticide use in the general community.

Barrhaven is the most successful example of multi-family, low-income housing for the environmentally hypersensitive built to date. The residents are reportedly happy with the apartments, both in terms of their increased health and well-being, and in terms of the quality of the construction.

The spartan appearance of the interiors is pleasantly rustic to some observers, while others find them uncomfortable. Even in the architect's view, there is perhaps too heavy a reliance on wood for someone with specific sensitivities to wood, though it hasn't been a problem with the residents to date.

One example of a technical difficulty resulting from the extreme health-conscious construction was that the elimination of synthetic plasticizers made the concrete ground-floor slab difficult to work, and consequently minor cracking occurred.

One expressed criticism is that the two-story apartments are potentially difficult to use for a person with debilitating sensitivities. One of the common symptoms of environmental hypersensitivity is dizziness and loss of strength and muscle control, which argues for designing for handicap accessibility as a general rule. This suggests marrying the concern for healthy building demonstrated here with the emerging field of "universal design"; designing to accommodate various age groups and states of mobility within the same structure.

SUMMARY TABLE

For Whom?

A range of environmentally hypersensitive occupants.

Climate and Site

Ottawa/Carleton Regional Municipality, Ontario, Canada. 45°N latitude, with temperatures ranging from 86°F (30°C) in summer to −15°F (−26°C) in winter.

The Building

A single, two-story structure, containing two one-bedroom apartments, three two-bedroom apartments and two three-bedroom apartments.

Design Emphasis

Exceptional standards of health and hygiene for low-income residents with environmental hypersensitivities.

Climatic Design—project relies on energy efficiency measures rather than climate-responsive orientation in order to fit the climate of Ontario. This is primarily due to severe budget and site constraints that precluded a more articulated plan. The compact plan is not optimal for daylight, with two of seven units having only one exposure and four of seven enjoying a southern exposure.

Energy Efficient Design (envelope systems)—superinsulated 2x8 frame construction over concrete block walls. Masonite exterior siding with a baked enamel finish (stucco was preferred but found too expensive). Argon-filled double glazing.

Resource Efficient Design—simple form and compact volume minimizes exterior envelope. Modular design based on concrete masonry unit dimension minimizes waste. Envelope assembly eliminates exterior sheathing (this was done to eliminate glue-based wood products.)

Air Quality Design—elimination of the construction cavities that can serve as mold and mildew reservoirs. Design to facilitate maintenance by providing complete access to all services, demountable ductwork for easy cleaning, all interior surfaces hard and easily cleaned. Air flow facilitated through strategic placement of both general supply and dedicated exhaust ports. Electric boiler and appliances rather than more energy efficient natural gas, fan-coil furnace to minimize fried dust. Heat recovery ventilator dismantled, washed and rebuilt with silicone rather than conventional foam rubber gaskets. Polypropylene core artificially aged by continuous high temperature operation before installation. Electrical services minimize the use of standard PVC sheathed cable by using surface conduits. All electrical wires contained within metal conduit. All fixtures either ceramic or metal rather than plastic. (The plastic smoke detector is the only exception to this rule.) The surface wiring conduits have the potential to be placed under negative pressure and exhausted to mechanical rooms if required by individual sensitivities.

Design for Isolation of Pollutants—zoning of plan from dirty to clean; vestibule is ample enough to leave street clothes. Storage opens onto public spaces rather than bedrooms. Glass cabinet with ducted exhaust provided for television and other potentially problematic personal belongings.

Design for Light—glazing omits use of low-emissivity coatings in favor of admitting a more complete spectrum of light.

Design for Noise Protection—the structure is placed at the rear of the site, remote from automobile traffic. Concrete block party walls provide high levels of acoustical separation between units. Two-story unit arrangement minimizes acoustical conflicts between floors.

Design for Low Maintenance—maintenance-free exterior materials (see below). Dense and durable interior materials with little or no finish to maintain.

Materials Selection

Foundations—poured in place concrete, free of air entrainment, plasticizers and other additives.

Frame—load-bearing concrete block party walls set in additive-free structural mortar, cores grouted solid. 2x8 wood stud framing bypassing floor structures and fixed to 2x4 bearers.

Roofing—prefinished metal roofing.

Exterior Finishes—hardboard exterior siding with baked enamel finish. Steel frames of porch assembly have baked enamel finish. Tongue-and-groove basswood planking. Foil-faced gypsum wall board, washed before installation to remove any rolling oil, with foil facing the interior and taped or caulked with 100% silicone to fully isolate contents of exterior envelope from the interior. Glued wood exterior sheathing omitted such that the insulation is contained only by the woven olefin air barrier. 1x3 strapping.

Insulation—rockwool blown insulation, omitting binders.

Windows and Doors—aluminum windows with baked enamel finish. Double pane glazing with argon gas fill.

Interior Finishes—concrete floors ground to expose aggregate and sealed with a nontoxic sodium silicate penetrating water repellent. Concrete block walls sealed with sodium silicate solution. Wood surfaces subject to wear finished with water-based urethane, other wood surfaces finished with water-based acrylic sealer. Concrete plank ceiling of first floor painted with zero VOCs acrylic paint.

Kitchen Cabinets—open wooden shelves and provisions for roll-out metal cabinets provided.

Heating, Air Conditioning, Air Filtration and Ventilation

Heating and A/C Type—wall hung electric boiler, ducted forced air with fan coil. Conduit in place for future addition of air conditioning systems.

Ventilation System Type—heat recovery ventilator ducted into fan coil. Exhaust from kitchen, washrooms, customizable filter bank. Air circulation fans mounted outside of air stream to avoid offgassing into supply air. Space provided for central vacuum system with exhaust ports provided on leeward side of building. Galvanized metal ductwork washed with mild muriatic acid solution to remove rolling oil before installation.

CASE STUDY 4
Remodeled Detached Home: Total Home Remodel and Additions

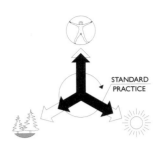

STANDARD
PRACTICE

Name: Craftsman home; Total home remodel and additions

Location: Olympia, Washington, Pacific Northwest coast

The owners are health care professionals with a young child. They have some allergies but no severe sensitivities. They bought the 1920s Craftsman-style cottage with many period features, with the intention to remodel it. They bought it for its charming character knowing that it was in poor condition and would require a significant investment of time and money. The owners are keenly aware of health problems related to poor indoor air quality through their medical practices, so the major goal of the remodel was to create a healthy home with an emphasis on prevention and light and air while still preserving the unique character of the house and adding some new rooms.

DESIGN PROCESS

The couple hired an architect who was sensitive to the unique character of the house and consultants who provided the healthy building input to the design. They researched materials, and hired a heating and ventilation consultant. The home required airlock entries, low-toxicity interiors, a lot of daylight in response to the northwest climate, reduced electromagnetic fields, and advanced heating and ventilation. Some of the rooms of the original plan were inadequate, so it was decided from the beginning that additions would be made, but these had to closely fit the style of the house. All design decisions were based on the usual criteria: personal taste, preserving the house style and keeping it affordable but, in addition, on elimination of pollution sources in the structure and mechanical and electrical systems. This meant that each decision had to be investigated to find out if healthy materials and systems would be feasible and affordable.

Large windows were chosen to provide ample daylight to every room, as well as cross-ventilation when needed. In an effort to reduce outside pollu-

Design Team: Liliane Bartha, Craig Southwell (consultants); Healthy Habitats; Dan Morris, Healthy Buildings Associates (Heating and Ventilating)
Architect: Kenneth Brooks

94

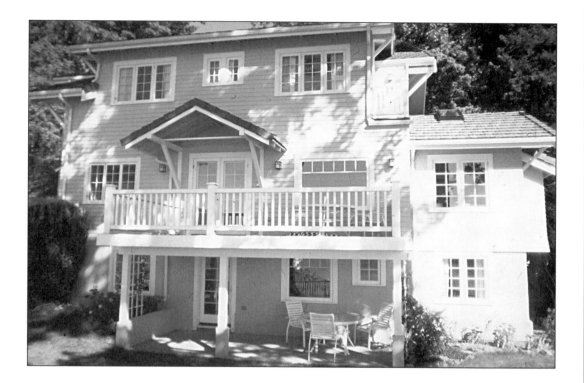

tion, such as pollens, both main and utility room entries were built as air locks with two doors.

It was decided to build the garage as a detached unit in order to keep car fumes and other odors from the indoor environment. A drainage system was installed to keep water from pooling around the house, potentially causing moisture damage during heavy rains. Landscaping was designed using locally adapted species and organic methods.

Insulation and draft sealing were brought up to current standards, all materials were carefully chosen for a low toxicity, and mechanical systems were designed for high ventilation and filtration efficiency. Electrical wiring was located to reduce field exposure.

Preserving the Craftsman character of this home was a major emphasis in the healthy remodel.

MATERIALS SELECTION

The consultants researched all materials, and collected samples and Material Safety Data Sheets (MSDS). A specialized air quality consultant was used periodically to resolve difficult choices. In order to keep the house free of plastics and adhesive materials, it was decided to use only solid wood and ceramic tile floors, low-toxicity finishes on floors and walls, no particle board or interior-grade plywood. The cabinets are solid wood with some

95

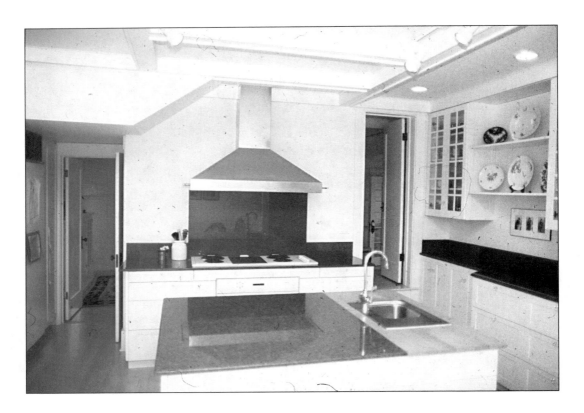

The kitchen is open, bright and cooking surfaces well ventilated and easily cleaned.

nonurea-formaldehyde MDF (medium density fiberboard) to natural stone counters, and untreated wood for windows and decks. Cotton insulation was used in new construction areas, and in the parts of the house that were gutted down to wood studs. A cementitious, sprayed-in-place insulation product was considered, but was not suited to the renovation project because its high moisture content can cause damage to existing wood and plaster construction during its lengthy drying process. An airtight drywall method was used for draft sealing gutted areas, as well as areas of new construction, using gasketed gypsum board to ensure as little air infiltration as possible. A low–vapor permeability, water-based sealer on the gypsum board was chosen as a vapor barrier, instead of polyethylene sheet which outgases and requires caulking and taping. A polyester (spunbonded polyolefin) weather barrier was installed as underlay for the concrete roofing tiles instead of the usual asphalt felt material ,which emits odorous tar compounds in warm weather.

MECHANICAL SYSTEMS

A heat pump with a fan coil was chosen for heating, with a gas water heater for domestic hot water. Continuous fan operation in the air handler, and both carbon and high-efficiency particulate filtration ensure that intake air and air recirculated in the home is kept thoroughly dust and odor free. A radiant heat system with a separate ventilation system would have been preferred, but it was not practical in the remodeled part of the home because it would have required totally new floors. The owners wanted control of the furnace air intake to allow slight pressurization on demand, to reduce entry of periodic wood smoke during winter.

Ventilation is provided by an outside air supply ducted into the fan coil just before the filters, so this exterior air supply was separately controlled by a damper to positively pressurize the house. An air-to-air heat exchanger was not installed due to space limitation and cost, but this would have been the consultants' recommendation for new construction. Supply registers were positioned to maximize delivery of air to the occupied zone in rooms. Returns were placed in the kitchen, hallway, bedrooms, bathrooms and some closets. All heating and ventilation ducts were washed before installation to remove oily residue from manufacturing. Exhaust fans were located over the kitchen cooktop, in all bathrooms and in the utility room to remove air contaminants. The kitchen cooktop exhaust is a large-capacity unit which could have depressurized the house, making air quality control difficult, so a fresh air supply fan is connected to the range and operates when the exhaust is on.

An isolated mechanical room was included in the addition which houses the water heater, ventilation/heating unit and central vacuum. The mechanical room has a separate exhaust and outside air supply. The electrical panels are also located in the room so electromagnetic field exposure is reduced in the occupied rooms. The original 1920s "knob and tube" wiring was replaced with steel-jacketed cable to minimize electrical fields. Ground fault interrupters were installed on the bedroom circuits to provide an opportunity to further reduce exposure by cutting off current at night.

The whole, original, galvanized steel plumbing system was replaced with copper pipes with lead-free solder. A whole house water filtration unit was installed, which incorporates a calcium carbonate (limestone) buffer to decrease leaching of copper due to the acidity of the municipal water supply. A reverse osmosis system under the kitchen sink provides drinking and cooking water.

CONSTRUCTION AND SUPERVISION

In 1992, when this project was in the planning stage, no contractor could be found locally who had experience building healthier homes. The owners interviewed 15 contractors, showing them drawings and specifications, but none had healthy building experience, and all were alarmed by the project. Consequently, the prices they quoted were very high, compared to conventional remodels. The couple eventually hired a contractor to do the renovation who said he was interested in the nontoxic aspect of the job, but he quit after five months at a particularly critical time. The roof had been taken off before a material had been chosen for a new one and the couple frequently had to visit the site late at night to prevent water damage. The contractor had also spilled gasoline on the gravel drive from his truck.

The owners then became their own contractors in what turned out to be an 18-month project. Delays were due to slow decision-making as well as to difficulty finding subcontractors willing to work with unusual materials and techniques. Finding trades who understood what the owners were trying to accomplish was very difficult. Many felt the specifications were too exacting, and took requests to do things differently as a negative comment on their skills. The job was finally completed, but it entailed a great deal of work for the owners.

STAR DIAGRAM ASSESSMENT AND CRITIQUE

Overall, the owners are happy with a home that maintains the flavor of the craftsman era, and supplies ample light and clean air to the occupants. They would have liked more durable coating on the hardwood floors and cabinets, and the one-part urethane floor system and cabinet finishes (painted and sealed with water-based lacquer) have not stood up well to a toddler's activities. More durable, low-toxicity products, such as the two-part cross-linked urethanes, will be used if refinishing is required. Landscaping is not yet finished and the glass storage system for filtered water in the kitchen still needs to be completed.

The results are excellent, but the process was difficult because the owners were not experienced project managers and there were numerous unanticipated costs and problems. The project was very expensive, even for a heritage remodel largely due to unforeseen problems and delays rather than the healthier building materials and methods. The owners' advice to anyone attempting a healthy building renovation is to hire a contractor with experience building in this fashion, build new if you have serious doubts about the renovation, and take a very deep breath! It will be a difficult experience, no matter how well prepared you are.

THE SUMMARY TABLE

For Whom?

A young professional couple with a small child. None has extreme health problems, but prevention is paramount.

Climate and Site

An older urban, single-family neighborhood in the Pacific northwest. Local streets are quiet, residential only, and there is no industry or agriculture nearby.

The Building

3600 sq. ft. (335 sq.m.) with additions. Detached two-car garage, entry, living room/dining room, parlor, kitchen, utility, three bathrooms, three bedrooms, office and guest room, separate mechanical room, plus a self-contained suite, one bedroom, living/dining room, kitchen, one bathroom and separate laundry.

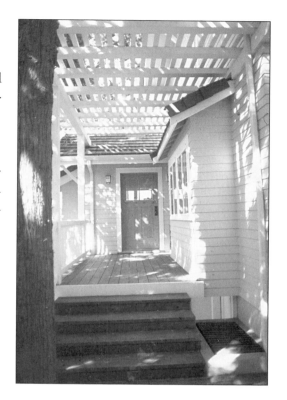

A sheltered entry appropriate to the coastal climate separates the garage from the house.

Design Emphasis

Daylight, sunlight, clean air, environmental control, maintaining the traditional charm and character of the home.

Climatic Design—daylight and maximum sunlight. Cross-ventilation.
Energy Efficient Design—upgraded insulation windows, and draft sealing for entire house. Heat pump furnace.
Resource Efficient Design—many parts of the old home were salvaged in the remodel.
Air Quality Design—low-toxicity materials, envelope air tightness, advanced ventilation and filtration, low-temperature heat.
Design for Isolation of Pollutants—separate mechanical room.
Design for Light—large new windows.
Design for EMF Protection—electrical panels located in isolated utility room, metallic sheathed type wiring was used to reduce field exposure.
Design for Low Maintenance—ceramic floors, built-in vacuum.
Other Design Emphasis—additions must fit the traditional character of the home.

Materials Selection

Foundations—additive-free concrete, metal termite shields.

Frame—standard wood frame with original part upgraded where necessary, plywood sheathing.

Roofing—concrete tile, polyolefin underlay.

Exterior Finishes—conventional paint, cedar siding.

Insulation—cotton batting insulation, airtight drywall method in retrofitted and new areas, low toxicity, vapor barrier primer.

Windows and Doors—wood sash, double glazed.

Interior Finishes—foil-clad gypsum board, low-toxicity acrylic sealer, zero VOCs paint.

Floor Coverings—slate and ceramic tile with no sealer in thinset mortar, maple and fir plank, one-part urethane finish.

Cabinets—formaldehyde-free particle board, paint and lacquer finishes (water-dispersed lacquer).

Furnishings—Persian rugs, certified organic cotton futon beds and cotton drapery and upholstery fabric, antique solid wood, new solid wood beds.

Heating, Air Conditioning, Air Filtration and Ventilation

Heating, A/C Type—air source heat pump with fan coil, in isolated utility room. Air intake with adjustment, bath and kitchen exhausts, two fireplaces (old fireplaces relined with heat-form units).

Ventilation System Type—adjustable makeup air ducted to fan coil. Exhaust fans in baths, utility and kitchen.

Filtration System Type—carbon and high-efficiency particulate filters (HEPA) in fan coil.

Other Mechanical Notes—makeup supply air fan to kitchen range to balance exhaust. Whole house carbon water filter with calcium carbonate buffer, plus reverse osmosis kitchen unit with carbon filter and glass storage vessels. Built-in vacuum with outside exhaust.

CASE STUDY 5
Remodeled Detached Home

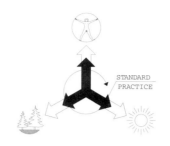

STANDARD PRACTICE

Name: Major Home Remodel.

Location: Sonoma County, California, temperate, dry

The family have a strong interest in natural, healthy living. No one in the family suffers from sensitivities, but they are concerned with prevention. This couple and their three children live on a small acreage north of the San Francisco Bay Area in an old farming community. They bought the 1920s bungalow intending to remodel it. The original kitchen was awkward and dark and they wanted a country kitchen and seating area which would become a new center for their home. It had to be spacious, bright and airy and they wanted to emphasize natural textures and colors.

DESIGN PROCESS

The home is a simple rectangle with a small side wing. It had been built and added to in an unplanned way. The rooflines were confused and poorly matched, the exterior materials were a mixture of wood siding and old shingles, and the windows were small and poorly placed. The interior spaces had been divided in an awkward way and there was no adequate seating area. Another problem was that the home was deteriorating due to poor foundations. Before the remodel, the owners had the building lifted and placed on a new concrete foundation because the old supports were rotting.

The owners hired an architect, Carol Venolia, with a reputation for healthy design and the use of natural materials. Carol used questionnaires, photos, lifestyle questions and materials samples to find out the family's preferences and needs. The family originally wanted to add 1000 square feet (93 square meters) to the home but they were restricted because of septic requirements. The plan to build a second story was abandoned and they decided to gut and rebuild the existing kitchen and add a sitting room, deck and fireplace. They also decided to rebuild parts of the roof. The main design themes which emerged from the early sketches were: daylight and sun; the fireplace at the center; an open, generous

Design Team:
Carol Venolia, Architect, and the owners
Builder: Marc Boudart, Boudart Construction

101

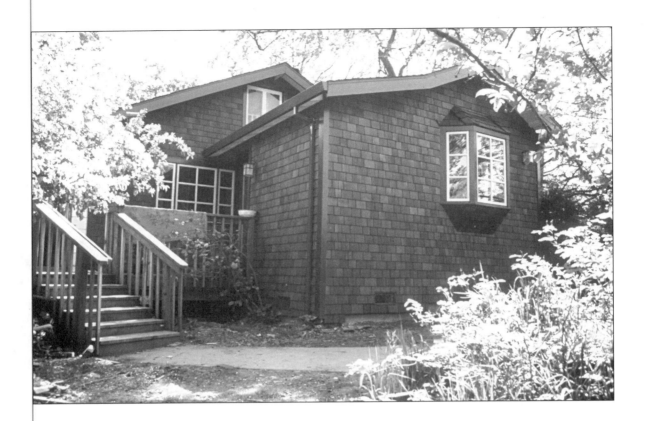

Remodeled home. The garden setting receives more emphasis than the modest exterior.

kitchen work area; and strong natural textures and colors. The kitchen was to have only lower cabinets and a work island, with the walls left free for windows. Air quality was not an explicit requirement, but was implicit in the emphasis on simple, natural interiors with few potential sources of pollution.

The builder was also part of the discussion from an early stage. He was chosen partly for his adobe experience because the design required curved forms in plaster. The builder is also a family friend who was enthusiastic about the idea of remodeling and restoring the old farmhouse using a natural design esthetic. He advised the owners on costs and some technical matters.

The final design required completely gutting the kitchen and seating area of the home, rebuilding the roof in some areas to remove some poorly spliced rooflines, adding a new deck with French doors, adding a bay window and other new windows and a skylight to the kitchen area, building a new fireplace with built-in seating, and installing a ceramic tile floor and all new kitchen cabinets and appliances. A "California cooler" space for storing fruits and vegetables was also included on the north wall, vented to the outdoors. In the process, it was necessary to replace the roofing and much of the siding, and restore other interior finishes.

MATERIALS SELECTION

Materials selection was done with a strong preference for rustic, hand-made appearances, and simple finishes from natural plant and mineral sources. The assumption was that these would also be healthy materials. There was no specific testing done, but all material sources were researched, and samples obtained. Materials were examined on site. For instance, the plaster was tinted and experimentally applied in a closet until the desired "inside of a sea shell" effect was achieved. Many other material decisions were made to match the existing construction or deal with needed repairs when problems were uncovered with the original construction. The owners rejected all typical options such as fiberglass and cellulose insulation. They then researched options such as wool, cotton, foamed silicates and foil-coated plastic bubble sheet, with the assistance of their architect.

MECHANICAL SYSTEMS

The existing gas space heater in the home was retained. The fireplace provides some heat, and a high-capacity kitchen exhaust was added for the commercial range.

The shallow well is easily contaminated. The previous owners had put a chlorinator in and the new owners removed it and added a filter and

The interior reflects thick walls, columns and small windows in the southwest adobe style which is appropriate to the California climate.

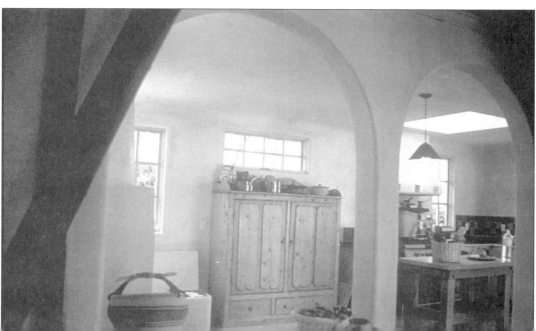

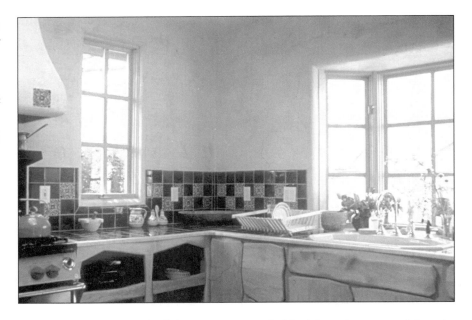

The kitchen is a unique result of a design collaboration with the cabinet maker and the owners' natural material selections.

ultraviolet sterilizer, which has proven unreliable. There is too much iron in the water and it clogs up the filter and sterilizer, and could be unsafe. The family has now drilled a new well which is protected from contamination.

CONSTRUCTION AND SUPERVISION

The contractor was chosen for his enthusiasm and support for the project from the beginning. As a family friend, the owners felt they could trust him and work closely with him. The architect provided the concept and basic working drawings, and was retained for code and design issues, but not for site review during construction. She was consulted over some decisions and helped with problem resolution during construction. The construction contract was not put to open bidding; the contractor provided a cost estimate. No formal specifications were used; many decisions about materials and details were made during the construction process.

The owners were fully involved in the remodel process and lived in part of the house during construction. Their living space was separated by plastic sheets from the construction area. They expedited materials and discussed details directly with the builder so decisions were made quickly. The project generally went very well, due to excellent communication and quick responses to any problems because there was someone home most of the time.

The major construction dilemma was that many detail and finishing decisions were made in progress, and not accurately priced, and so a budget could not be closely followed. This resulted in costs which stretched far beyond original expectations. But the work and details also stretched far beyond what was originally anticipated. For example, the cabinets were designed and built from solid hardwood by a cabinetmaker who worked directly with the owners and coordinated with the builder. The results are unique, and could not have been easily anticipated or priced.

Another major obstacle was the foil/plastic bubble sheet finally chosen for insulation. The inspector wouldn't accept it because it did not have a direct equivalency to the insulation requirement under the California Energy Code. The manufacturer provided data but the inspector insisted that it still wasn't considered an equivalent under code. The problem was finally resolved after some occasionally acrimonious discussion, mediated by the architect, between the manufacturer and the building department. After the insulation was finally accepted, four layers were used for the walls. The builder enjoyed handling it because there was no fiber, no odor and no problem with waste.

A lot of substandard work in the older parts was uncovered which had to be upgraded—the old rooflines were straightened out and minor rot was removed. The wood forms behind the curved plaster were complex and the builder's experience with adobe was very helpful.

The cost was very high on a square-foot basis due to the poor condition of the old house and labor-intensive finishing.

STAR DIAGRAM ASSESSMENT AND CRITIQUE

The owners are delighted with the outcome and feel that they finally have the farm kitchen and seating area that their small home needed. Though no special health emphasis was identified, the health benefit is implicit in the whole approach. The results feel unique, comfortable and fitting to family life in the country. The main health problem was poor water quality. Treating the contaminated well did not work and a new well was necessary. The owners are also planning to replace the furnace, which they do not find satisfactory. Resource efficiency was not emphasized except through salvaging existing construction. Energy efficiency is not extraordinary beyond what is required by California law, but is aided by the California cooler, which reduces refrigeration needs, and the use of passive solar heat and daylight to reduce space heating and lighting requirements.

THE SUMMARY TABLE

For Whom?

A family with three children at home.

Climate and Site

The climate is temperate, northern California coastal, approx. 20 in. (400 mm) annual precipitation, 40°F (4°C) winter low, 100°F (38°C) summer high. Three-acre agricultural lot in a semi-rural area, distant from highways and industry. Relatively flat site with adequate drainage, some heavy clay soils and serious termite problems.

The Building

1920s home, 1000 sq. ft. (93 sq.m.), living room, dining room, kitchen/ sitting room, bathroom, bedroom, loft.

Design Emphasis

Climatic Design—optimizes solar access, daylight and cross-ventilation. Uses outdoor air for food storage (California cooler).

Energy Efficient Design—insulation and thermal windows to California Energy Code Standards.

Resource Efficient Design—reclaimed much of the original construction.

Air Quality Design—natural materials selection, safe paints and sealers, natural ventilation.

Design for Light—generous clear glass areas, skylight, light interior finishes.

Design for Noise Protection—no special effort

Design for EMF field protection—no special effort.

Design for Low Maintenance—ceramic floors, hard plaster surfaces.

Other Design Emphasis—natural shapes, minimal square corners.

Materials Selection

Foundations—new, concrete perimeter, no special termite or rot protection.

Frame—conventional wood frame with redwood sills, 2x4 wood walls, 2x10 floor joists, plywood sheathing and subfloors.

Roofing—post and beam roof, fiber cement shingles.

Exterior Finishes—redwood siding and cedar shingles in natural stain, all-natural oil sealer.

Insulation—four layers of polyethylene foil bubble pack with air spaces.

Windows and Doors—solid wood doors and window sash, double glazed.

Interior Finishes—tongue and groove redwood paneling, exposed beams, tinted gypsum three-coat plaster on expanded metal lath for ceilings and walls, mineral color additive, all-natural, low-toxicity paints and sealers.

Floor Coverings—heavy ceramic tile in mortar bed, cement grout, all-natural sealer, some old fir floors.

Cabinets—solid hardwood, all-natural stains and sealers, countertops of Tunisian tile.

Furnishings—antiques, solid wood, built-in cement plaster furniture.

Heating, Air Conditioning, Air Filtration and Ventilation

Heating, A/C Type—single, free-standing gas space heater, fireplace which provides nominal heat

Ventilation System Type—high-capacity exhaust hood for commercial kitchen range

Water—shallow well is easily contaminated, required a new well.

Other Mechanical Notes—California cooler cabinet vented to north side.

CASE STUDY 6
New Duplex, Toronto Healthy House

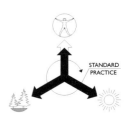

STANDARD PRACTICE

Design Team:
Martin Liefhebber, Architect; RAL Engineering; Waterloo Biofilter Systems Inc.; Doug Hart (solar design); Per Drewes (electrical systems); Blue Heron Environmental Technology; Ed Lowans (healthy materials)

Builder: Rolf Paloheimo, Creative Communities Research Inc.

Technical Assistance and Communications:
Christopher Ives, Debra Wright, Canada Mortgage and Housing Corp.

Name: Toronto Healthy House, new home

Location: Southern Great Lakes, Toronto, Ontario, cold climate.

Winner of the 1992 Canadian Mortgage and Housing Corporation Healthy Home Design Competition, the Toronto Healthy House is the first energy and water self-sufficient demonstration house incorporating healthy building practices built in a Canadian city. The design competition used a broad definition of healthy buildings, that included intensive urban land use, energy and water conservation, materials resource efficiency, indoor air quality and affordability. The urban duplex project is an "infill design," meaning that it adds new housing to existing building lots without demolitions. Infills typically do not require new subdivisions, new road construction or new utility construction.

Each unit in the duplex is 1700 square feet (158 square meters) on four levels, with a common wall at the center. They are unconnected to sewers, water or gas, and only one of the two units is connected to city electricity. Both have large rainwater collection systems, biological wastewater treatment and recycling systems, solar water heaters and large photovoltaic panels. One unit has a battery storage system for the photovoltaic electricity; the other is connected to the city's electric system so that the owner receives credits for the power generated by the panels (to offset their purchased electricity bill). The units produce about 75% of their own energy from solar, and use about 80% recycled water. The units are super energy-efficient, have non-toxic materials indoors, highly effective ventilation and heating, and receive generous daylight and sunlight, while shading excess summer sun.

DESIGN PROCESS

Because the project is for demonstration, it incorporates many unusual features. However, it also had to be affordable and practical to build and live in. It was to be as independent of utilities as possible, but the technologies used had to be well proven.

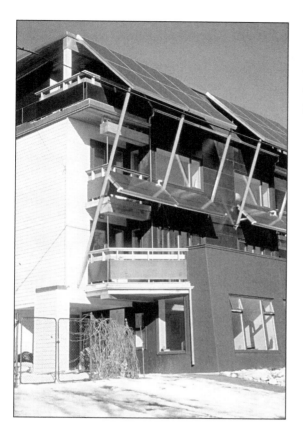

Southeast view, showing street entrance, very compact carport and balconies above, shaded by photovoltaic panels.

Initially, the architect proposed building a very compact (800 square feet or 75 square meters) duplex, with each unit incorporating a solar greenhouse with a built-in biological wastewater treatment system. Because it was to be an infill, the plan required that the architect find an existing lot in a built-up area, but this was difficult because an infill site is often very controversial in a neighborhood. Many municipal areas do not want more housing built inside their existing developed areas. Finally, after three years, a 45- x 71-foot (14- x 22-meter) lot on a steep slope facing south was found. The lot is actually the rear yards of two existing older homes on the higher ground, which didn't have the usual garage behind them. The lot had no sewer, water or gas, and would have cost over $110,000 US to connect, which is why it hadn't been developed before.

Once the site was found, an experienced developer/builder was located who not only wished to build it, but would live in one of the units and sell the other. The original compact design (for which the architect won the design award) was modified to more closely meet market expectations. It was enlarged to 1700-square-foot (158-square meter) units, with master bed-

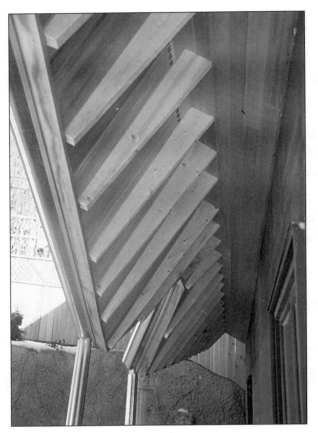

rooms and ensuite baths on top. The greenhouse in the original design was discarded in favor of an enclosed wastewater treatment system which requires little maintenance and takes little floor space.

One design principle emphasized was that as many features as possible had to serve multiple functions. For example, the solar panels not only produce electricity and hot water, but they also shade the south wall from excessive sun. The upper floors are concrete slabs for thermal storage of direct solar heat, and they are further heated by circulating hot water from solar collectors and wastewater heat recovery. The corrugated, galvanized steel forms for these slabs are simply painted on the underside to provide the ceiling finish below. The top surface of the concrete is polished and sealed to provide a finished floor.

Soffit details showing engineered wood components used throughout this resource efficient home.

The healthy building features of the duplex are based on low-toxicity materials, and effective ventilation and heating. Daylight and solar features make the interiors bright and attractive, without excessive dependence on electric lighting. The water quality is independent of municipal water, because municipal water is not used. Instead, collected rainwater for drinking is sterilized, using ultraviolet light. Sand barriers rather than toxic soil treatments were used to keep termites away from the foundation.

Because energy efficiency is a primary goal for a self-sufficient home, passive solar design, superinsulated walls and roof, and high performance windows were important energy design strategies. The units are designed to maximize passive solar use through careful positioning of windows, thermal mass storage (primarily in the floors), active thermal storage (in the water heating system) and designing for natural ventilation. The open stairwell, large doors and operable windows on each level allow natural ventilation and cooling. In summer, heated air exits through the upper openings, drawing cooler air in from the ground-level openings. Both the solar

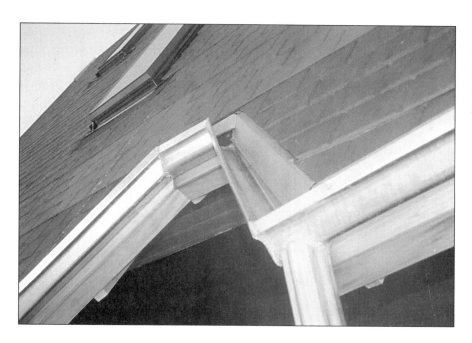

Part of the rainwater and snow-melt collection system.

panels and landscaping are placed to provide summer shading. The rainwater collection and storage system and wastewater recycling systems provide for most household water. Each unit relies primarily on rain and snow feeding into a 5,000-gallon (20,000-liter) storage tank for its water supply. Collected water is filtered and sterilized for potable use. Ultra-low-consumption fixtures reduce water use, and wastewater is treated with a biological filter system and recirculated for washing, flushing, bathing and gardening.

The materials used in construction were carefully selected for their resource and energy efficiency, and low toxicity. For example, the wall framing was done with manufactured "I" section studs (usually used for floor joists),

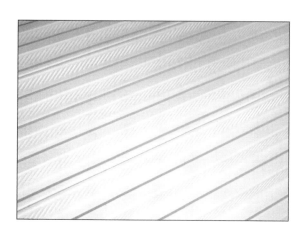

The steel forms for the concrete floors have been painted with a low toxicity paint to form the ceilings below.

111

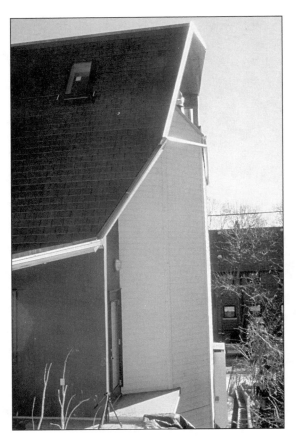

West wall.

because they are made from fast-growing, small-diameter trees, and allow for nine inches of wall insulation while reducing thermal bridging (heat transfer through conductive framing members). The foundation walls were formed with a hollow block made with recycled wood scraps and cement. The cores of the blocks were filled with concrete and reinforcing steel, and the outside face of the blocks insulated with a rigid mineral fiber board. The siding is a combination of very durable fiber-cement panels and weather-resistant, resin-saturated plywood.

An airtight drywall system was used for the walls and top-level ceiling to ensure good containment of the insulation, minimal air leakage and excellent moisture control, and to prevent outdoor pollutants entering from air leaks. The wall system is independent of the structural concrete floors (to minimize leaky seams), and was tested with a house pressurization fan to ensure its integrity. The insulation is mineral wool, chosen because it contains no resin binders, and because it is made primarily from wastes (slag) from mineral processing.

The wastewater treatment system was a major design challenge, and proved difficult to get approved by health authorities. The system recycles wastewater for the laundry, bath and toilets using an anaerobic tank, settling tanks, gravel and sand filters, and an aerobic biological reactor. The treated water then circulates twice through an ultraviolet sterilizer and then a sand and activated carbon filter before being used for washing and flushing. The drinking water from the underground storage cistern passes through sand filters and is then sterilized by a separate ultraviolet lamp before use.

The electrical system was another major design challenge. In one unit, photovoltaic panels charge batteries which supply an inverter to convert it to standard house current. The lighting, refrigeration, kitchen appliances and all pumps and motors have been carefully selected or custom built to conserve electricity. There is no electric clothes dryer, but there is a clothes drying cabinet with an air supply heated by waste heat recovered from the building ex-

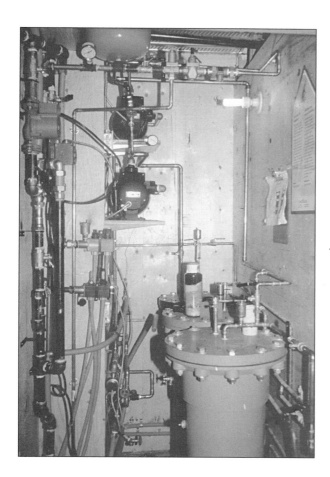

The central mechanical
room is the heart of the
water systems and
heating (upper left).

Graded sand and gravel
are used to filter
rainwater and recycled
waste water (below left).

A reflective light collector
funnels light into the
stairwell (below right).

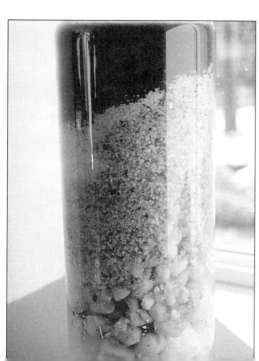

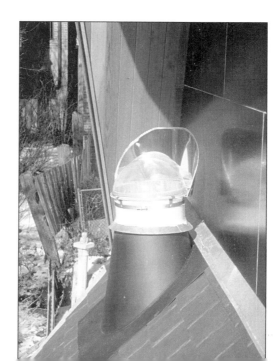

haust. This unit is not supplied by the electrical utility. The other unit has its photovoltaic panels connected to an inverter and controller which is connected to the electrical utility. When the house uses more electricity than the panels generate (at night, for example), the energy is purchased from the utility. When the house generates more than it uses, the surplus is fed into the utility and the meter credits the owners, up to a zero balance.

The architectural expression of these advanced, healthy building features is very eclectic and contemporary, emphasizing bold colors and unadorned surfaces. It has an almost industrial look, making very little reference to traditional housing types in the city. The architect chose to make a statement that these houses represent the future, and so should look and feel nontraditonal. Though they look different, they are pleasant and comfortable to live in, and do not require special expertise or dramatic lifestyle changes.

MATERIALS SELECTION

The architect and a healthy materials consultant chose materials based on recycled content, low toxicity, durability and resource efficiency. Extensive

The battery storage system for the "off-grid" house.

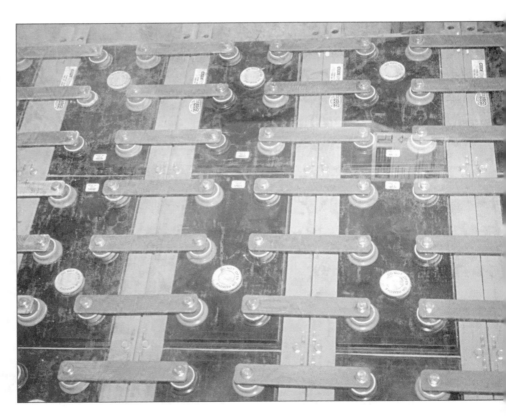

research was done using resource guides and by contacting manufacturers. There was no identifiable "user" because one of the units was going to be sold after completion, so healthy material choices were made on the basis of general knowledge, comparative research and reasonable caution. The project was not designed specifically for an environmentally hypersensitive occupant, but is expected to have very good indoor air quality.

All the wall and roof structural materials are manufactured wood products which are made from low-grade and waste woods, for resource efficiency.

MECHANICAL SYSTEMS

Radiant floor heat was chosen because it is healthy and can easily use the varied water temperatures provided by the solar water heaters. Water is heated by the collectors, and the hottest goes for washing and bathing. Slightly cooler water is circulated, on demand, for in-floor heating. The incoming water is preheated by a coil which extracts heat from the outgoing wastewater. Buried pipes also use the earth around the home to absorb heat in the summer (for indoor cooling), and to supplement solar heating in winter.

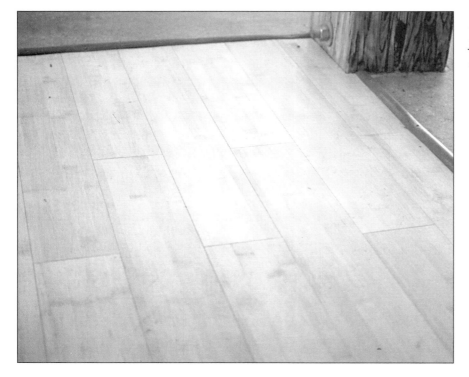

Flooring made from Asian bamboo.

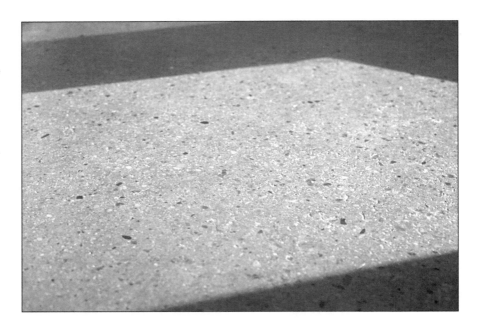

Most floors are polished and sealed concrete.

The ventilation system is based on a heat recovery ventilator with a metal core which extracts exhaust from the kitchen, baths, laundry and clothes drying cabinet. The heat is then transferred to the incoming air, which is filtered by a unique "turbulent flow precipitator," a device which extracts dust from the air by forcing the air stream past collection chambers. The cooled exhaust stream is then used to prevent freezing of the insulated outdoor compartment which houses a small, alcohol fueled standby generator. The generator coolant discharges heat into the home heating system (co-generation).

There is a central vacuum in a storage closet in the entry area. The European front-loading clothes washer is very energy and water efficient. The electric cooktop and refrigerator were custom built from the most energy efficient products available. The refrigerator uses a compressor with an electronically controlled motor which is mounted outdoors to cool more efficiently. The refrigerator cabinet uses a special vacuum insulation panel which is far more efficient than the best plastic or mineral insulations.

CONSTRUCTION AND SUPERVISION

The contractor is the developer and owner/occupant of one of the units. He has a strong interest in environmentally responsible construction, and secured many donations of materials and services which the project showcased.

The developer used his connections to trades and laborers, to bring in people who were highly motivated to learn from a new experience. Once a site was found, the project generally went very well, due to careful preparation and exacting management. The contractor had some difficulty with special materials and procedures, such as painting the galvanized steel ceilings with a low-toxicity paint, but the major construction dilemma resulted from the very tight time limits to get the project open for professional and public tours. Some items had to remain unfinished, and some had to be finished temporarily to meet deadlines. There were also difficulties gaining approvals for the unusual systems.

The Canada Mortgage and Housing Corporation provided technical support, technical management, and house monitoring and communications throughout the entire process. They have also operated the tours and are producing the publications describing the house.

Due to the special energy and resource efficient features, this project cost substantially more to build than a comparable custom home. However, some costs were offset by simplification of finishes, and many of these features will pay for themselves over time by reducing operating costs.

STAR DIAGRAM ASSESSMENT AND CRITIQUE

The project seems to be a very successful demonstration of independence from utilities, though it is too early to say how well all the systems will perform. For example, the wastewater treatment system will be tested regularly for a period of two years to determine its effectiveness in removing contaminants and bacteria. The enhanced indoor environment seems to be successful and the solar features performed well through the first winter. The major success of this project is its ability to educate and inspire visitors about a more sustainable urban future.

The design approach is in distinct contrast to the Vancouver Healthy Home. This house makes the solar panels very prominent, and uses unusual colors and roof lines to express its uniqueness. The Vancouver House uses traditional roof lines and colors to blend into the existing neighborhood. The houses demonstrate that healthy housing can be as as distinctive or as unobtrusive as wished.

THE SUMMARY TABLE

For Whom?

Built for demonstration and the market.

Climate and Site

The climate is southern Great Lakes, approx. 30 in. (760 mm) annual precipitation, –3°F (–20°C) winter low, 87°F (30°C) summer high. South slope with poorly drained clay soil. Moderate termite problems.

The Building

New construction, 1996. 2 x 1700 sq.ft. (158 sq.m.), 3 bedrooms, 2 1/2 baths, kitchen, dining room, living room, office/sun room. Attached single carport.

Design Emphasis

Climatic Design—maximizes solar exposure, daylight, stack ventilation and sun shelter.

Energy Efficient Design—the majority of space heating is provided by solar gain and storage. Thermal insulation and windows are very high performance. Carefully selected, low-consumption appliances are used throughout. The refrigerator has vacuum insulation and an external compressor. A clothes drying cabinet replaced a dryer. High-efficiency electric lighting and motors have been used throughout. A solar heater provides domestic hot water and some space heating. A ground loop provides heat storage in summer and some heating in winter. A photovoltaic and battery storage system provide the majority of electricity for the off-grid house. A fuel fired co-generator provides backup power. The grid-connected house has photovoltaics which feed surplus energy back into the power grid. A heat recovery ventilator is used.

Resource Efficient Design—many materials with recycled content were chosen. All wood products are manufactured from fast-growing species.

Air Quality Design—mechanical termite barriers (sand) are used instead of toxic soil treatments. Pollutant source control is achieved by using low-emission interior finishes. High ventilation effectiveness is achieved through ventilation system design and turbulent flow filtration. A radiant heating system in the concrete floors ensures minimal dust problems. High-performance insulation, windows and moisture control (through ventilation) minimize interior surface condensation to prevent mold growth.

Design for Light—rooms are shallow or open from front to back. They have large glass areas, and most have two exposures.

Design for Noise Protection—no special effort.

Design for EMF Protection—no special effort.

Design for Low Maintenance—concrete floors, built-in vacuum.
Other Design Emphasis—bright and contrasting colors.

Materials Selection

Foundations—cement-stabilized, wood fiber blocks with concrete fill.
Frame—nine in "I" section wood walls, cast concrete floors, fourteen in "I" section wood roof framing, insulating sheathing.
Roofing—rubber membrane, composition shingles.
Exterior Finishes—fiber cement and resin-saturated plywood panel siding.
Insulation—mineral wool board and batts, airtight drywall system.
Windows and Doors—fiberglass window sash, multiple glazed units with low-emission coating, argon fill and insulating spacers. Solid wood and hardboard panel interior doors.
Interior Finishes—standard gypsum board, low-toxicity sealer, zero VOCs paint, formaldehyde-free fiber board trims, clear sealer.
Floor Coverings—polished concrete sealed with waterglass (sodium silicate) sealer, birch, and laminated bamboo planks on stairs.
Cabinets—formaldehyde-free fiber board with clear sealer (no laminates or paints), mineral filled polyester composite and custom cast concrete countertops.
Other—all wall and roof structural materials are manufactured wood products, made from low-grade and waste woods. All upper floors are concrete slabs. This is a very unusual structure, because the concrete floors are supported on wood beams and columns.

Heating, Air Conditioning, Air Filtration and Ventilation

Heating, A/C Type—solar water heaters, hot water radiant slab heating.
Ventilation System Type—a heat recovery ventilator ducted to all rooms, exhausts in kitchen, laundry and clothes drying cabinet.
Filtration System Type—turbulent flow precipitator on ventilation air supply.
Other Mechanical Notes—built-in vacuum, rainwater and snowmelt collection and treatment system. Wastewater treatment and recycling system. Advanced photovoltaic system with battery storage or grid connection.

Oetzel House, New Home

STANDARD PRACTICE

Name: Oetzel House

Location: Near Austin, Texas, hot, humid climate

Mary Oetzel is a healthy building consultant whose expertise has been developed through both professional research and personal experience. She has consulted on the materials specification and construction practices of numerous houses, offices and schools, and is currently on a Texas State Health Department task force to establish voluntary indoor air quality standards for the state's public schools. She credits her self-designed house with helping her to regain her own health after years of chronic health problems associated with exposure to pesticides and other chemicals commonly found in home and work environments.

DESIGN PROCESS

Mary creates healthy housing by adapting conventional dwellings using careful materials selection and meticulous construction supervision. Outwardly, her house is a pleasant one-story ranch, typical for new construction in the region. Beneath the surface, however, nontoxic, low-maintenance ways of doing things have been substituted for more conventional solutions throughout. Her message to clients is that healthy housing need not stand out as different, but more care must go into its making and maintenance.

The desire for clean air determined both the site and siting of the house. The land is within commuting distance of Austin, Texas, but is relatively undeveloped. It is in a nonagricultural scrub forest, so there is little chance of exposure to agricultural or lawn chemicals. The house sits in the center of a 15-acre parcel, which further ensures clean air by providing a land buffer against nearby development. The land immediately surrounding the house has been cleared to facilitate air movement and to dry the ground, which cuts down on mold and reduces the risk of termites. This consequently reduces the need for insecticides. Within this clearing, the house is oriented to take advantage of the prevailing breeze for natural cooling.

Mary gave special attention to the problem of eliminating pesticides and

Design Team:
Mary Oetzel

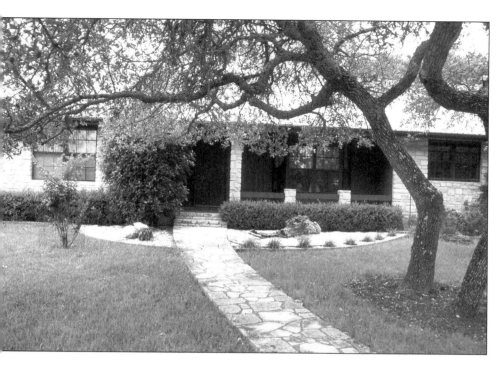

A healthy home can easily belong in its neighborhood without any exterior signs of its differences.

biocides, both inside and outside the house. As mentioned above, the brush around the house is cut back, creating a traditional lawn. The lawn is maintained with organic fertilizers but it does require mowing, which necessitates the house being shut to prevent exhaust fumes from entering. Still, the lawn ensures that the house and the immediate surroundings are as dry and well drained as possible in the hot and humid climate, controlling insect and moisture-related problems without the use of chemicals. Also in this vein, the slab of the house is elevated by a foot to guard against insect penetration at the sill. Finally, a carefully sealed vapor barrier plays a role in keeping insects out of the house, as does the use of diatomaceous earth, soap spray and good housekeeping habits.

MATERIALS SELECTION

The materials used for the house were chosen to satisfy several health criteria. They had to be pesticide and biocide free. They could not off-gas volatile organic compounds such as formaldehyde. They would need to be maintained with nontoxic practices, and so could not depend on constant repainting or resealing. The result in many ways is a return to pre–World War II construction technologies that don't rely on products of the chemical revolution. In this mild climate, the exclusion of questionable materi-

121

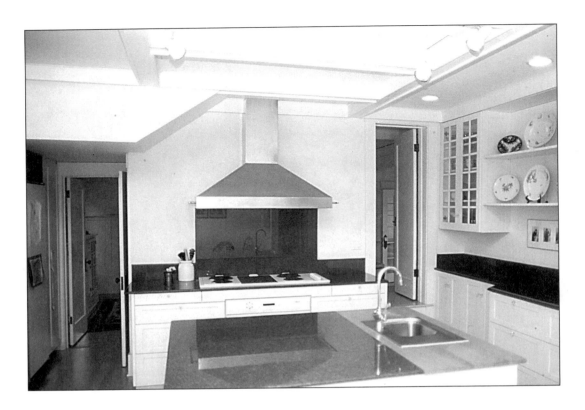

als such as adhesives and sealants did not pose the same challenges in terms of energy efficiency that other case studies examine. The healthy alternatives simply demanded a greater degree of craftsmanship from the builders.

The house is built using conventional wood framing on a concrete slab. Inside, the majority of the interior is finished in an elegant unpainted cement plaster without gypsum or chemical additives. The dense, smooth surfaces of these walls are still in very good condition after 16 years and are touched up if scuffed "with a little sandpaper."

As a healthy building consultant, Mary says the testing of materials to determine their specific acceptability to clients is the cornerstone of the materials selection process. Her advice is to try things out in small increments. For instance, she had one room plastered and lived with it for a week before deciding to use the plaster throughout the house. Mary's office is painted with an oil-based enamel to test a product that she was considering recommending. She found it quite acceptable once cured, though she no longer recommends it for extremely sensitive people because complete curing took over a year. In contrast, the utility and bathrooms are painted with custom-manufactured preservative-free latex paints.

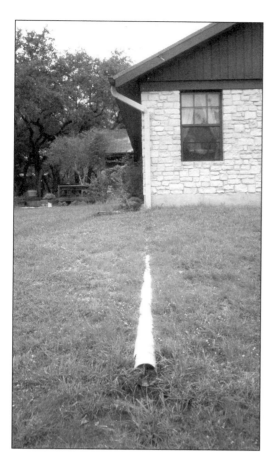

The site has been carefully cleared, sloped and drained to prevent moisture problems and minimize insect attacks.

The exterior of the house was painted with a custom-mixed biocide-free latex paint. This is a double-edged issue, however. In some situations mildew can be such a problem that Mary would recommend a conventional house paint while still seeking to minimize its presence in spaces close to human contact. Latex caulk was used on the exterior, but Mary no longer recommends this to her clients because of the biocides and mildewcides they contain. Rather, she would recommend paintable, 100% silicone caulk, which can be used both within the house and on the exterior.

MECHANICAL SYSTEMS

The house is cooled naturally, with air conditioning provided by a heat pump during the hottest months. Every room is designed for some sort of cross-ventilation, with operable windows on two or more walls. The cathedral ceiling helps to expand the airiness of the rooms, an effect enhanced

123

with ceiling fans. Finally, a whole house fan is used to ventilate the house when natural air movement is insufficient.

Winter heating is provided by a fan-coil unit connected to the heat pump. This is mounted centrally within the house to minimize ductwork. The unit's filter has been upgraded and the fiberglass lining removed, as has the lining of the ductwork, to ensure that fiberglass does not enter the air stream. The unit is noisy as a result and now Mary would suggest isolating the unit by suspending it from the attic rafters and increasing the duct size to allow for slower air movement.

CONSTRUCTION AND SUPERVISION

Mary's philosophy is that the process of building a "healthy" structure is more critical than its design. She advises having a person on site daily to catch problematic substitutions and unthinking contamination. During the construction of her own house such potentially contaminating activities as smoking and spraying for wasps were not allowed on the job site and gas-powered generators were kept outside of the house itself. The metal for the duct system, which typically arrives coated with machine oil, was taken to a car wash and thoroughly cleaned before installation.

STAR DIAGRAM ASSESSMENT AND CRITIQUE

The Oetzel house is a strong response to both health and energy efficiency issues. In addition to the climate-responsive features mentioned in relation to health, the windows include integral storm windows, the metal roof is vented and includes a radiant barrier, the west side of the house is completely shaded by trees, and the southern overhangs are designed to provide shade in the summer while allowing winter sun penetration. All of these features ensure that the house stays naturally comfortable year round. For further energy savings, the house is equipped with solar collectors that provide hot water for the shower and taps.

The house's remoteness and large lot ensure good ambient air quality, but represent a conflict between the goals of health and resource sustainability by implying dependence on an automobile. The house does not make use of engineered wood products or recycled content materials, though Mary does see a role for such things if they are thoroughly encapsulated, and the modest scale of her house is inherently resource conserving. Mary is extremely happy with her house, both for its high standard of indoor air quality and for the comfortable setting it provides.

SUMMARY TABLE

For Whom?

A healthy building consultant with chemical sensitivities.

Climate and Site

The climate is mild, conducive to natural ventilation and outdoor living. The house is centered on a large lot in a rural nonagricultural subdivision. The cleared site lowers humidity levels, increases ventilation and controls insect breeding grounds.

The Building

1924 sq.ft. (180 sq.m.) single family house in the rural hill country of Texas (1980). Single-story slab on grade construction.

Design Emphasis

Climatic Design—cathedral ceiling promotes ventilation in hot weather. Screened-in porch allows for indoor/outdoor living, expanding the usable area of the house. The house is oriented five degrees east of south to front the prevailing breeze, which also works well for sun shading. Every room has cross-ventilation.

Energy Efficient Design (envelope systems)—vented metal roof with radiant barrier. A carefully constructed vapor barrier provides both good indoor air quality and energy efficiency. The house is well insulated for the mild climate, with both fiberglass batts and rigid fiberglass sheathing.

Air Quality Design—elimination of all construction materials containing offgassing chemicals, formaldehyde, pesticides and biocides. Envelope design to control moisture movement that could produce mold. Electric as opposed to natural gas appliances to avoid combustion within the house. No caulk used indoors except for the basket strainers in the sink, and here 100% silicone is used. The bathroom basins are set into grout. No paint used except in the office, utility and bathrooms. To minimize presence of plastics in the house, all of the potable water plumbing uses copper piping with acid- and lead-free solder. The wastewater lines are copper within the house and PVC within the concrete slab.

Design for Isolation of Pollutants—the joints between foil-faced batts were taped to create a continuous vapor barrier. This controls moisture migration and resulting potential for mold problems as well as containing potential indoor air contaminants within the envelope assembly. Mary now recommends using either a high-density polyethylene or construction-grade aluminum foil as a vapor barrier. All electrical wiring contained in conduit.

Design for Light— the roof and landscaping are designed to provide summer shade while allowing winter sun penetration.

Design for Noise Protection—remote site.

Design for EMF Protection—this was not something that was addressed when the house was built. Since then, the house has been tested several times and does not show any unusual electromagnetic field levels.

Design for Low Maintenance—brick exterior cladding, landscaping contains minimal shrubbery, design has a simple plan, simple details, all hard surfaces, minimal drapery and washable upholstery and throw rugs.

Materials Selection

Foundations—additive-free concrete slab raised above grade.

Frame—conventional wood stud construction. No plywood or particle board used for sheathing.

Roofing—unpainted galvanized metal.

Exterior Finishes—locally available stone, solid wood trim, custom-mixed latex paint without biocides or mildewcides.

Insulation—foil-faced fiberglass batts. Compressed fiberglass nonstructural sheathing board behind stone facing and pesticide-free, foil-faced compressed cardboard behind wood siding.

Windows and Doors—metal window frames with integral storm windows. Metal exterior doors and six-panel solid wood interior doors.

Interior Finishes—most walls and ceilings unpainted traditional cement plaster with no chemical additives. Office is painted with an oil-based enamel. Utility and bathrooms painted with custom biocide-free latex.

Floor Coverings—glazed ceramic tile floor in thickset Portland cement mortar on concrete slab. Site-mixed Portland cement and sand used as grout.

Kitchen Cabinets—countertop: ceramic tile in thickset mortar (Portland cement, sand and water). Grout: commercial Portland cement grout without latex modifiers. The grout was water cured (kept wet for 15 days) which aids in the hydration of the cement and adds strength. Cabinets are solid oak and are constructed without backs, avoiding the use of pressed wood products.

Furnishings—minimal use of drapery to avoid creating dust sinks. Furniture all reupholstered with organic cotton and all coil-spring construction without upholstery foam. Easily washable cotton area rugs.

Other—the house is designed with special regard to controlling insect attack without the use of pesticides. The site is cleared to dry the land, the house has French drains that take rainwater away from the house, the slab is raised 12 inches above grade to discourage termite attack, and the vapor barrier under the concrete slab serves as much to control insect movement as it does to control moisture movement.

Heating, Air Conditioning, Air Filtration and Ventilation

Heating, A/C Type—centrally located heat pump and fan-coil unit. The heat pump's fiberglass lining has been removed to avoid fiberglass contamination. All metal ducts without acoustical liners. The ducts were washed before installation.

Ventilation System Types—natural cross-flow ventilation through operable windows, supplemented by ceiling fans and a whole house fan. Range hood and bathrooms have exhaust fans.

Filtration System Type—electrostatically charged passive filter. All potable water is bottled due to poor-quality well water. Conventional chlorinator, carbon filter and softener used on domestic supply.

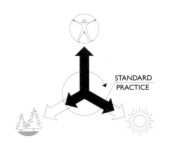

C A S E   S T U D Y   8

Pitman Residence, New Home

STANDARD PRACTICE

Name: The Pitman House

Location: Wimberley, Texas, hot, humid climate.

Sue Pitman and her children first began to have problems with their health the winter after moving into a new, tightly sealed suburban house in the Lake Bluff area of Chicago in 1977. A second house in the same area proved better, but a second factor, the neighborhood's heavy use of lawn pesticides, began to appear connected to the family's health problems. In 1984 Sue's husband's work shifted to Austin, Texas, and the family built the first of two homes in the nearby resort community of Wimberley. The house shown here is the Pitman's second, built in 1986. It sits on the same property as the first house, which is now rented out to others with chemical sensitivities.

The Hill Country is known in Texas as a retreat from extremes of heat and humidity. The landscape features rolling hills of rocky soils, covered with grasses, live oak and cedar. Wimberley in particular is home to the largest community of people with environmental hypersensitivities in the United States. The climate allows almost year-round outdoor living for people who have difficulty finding healthy enclosed environments, and the landscape is unproductive agriculturally and so free of potential exposure to agricultural pesticides.

The two houses are on a private 10-acre lot in a subdivision surrounded by working ranches. The roads in the neighborhood are dirt rather than asphalt, which suits the Pitmans' health needs. The landscape does produce a great deal of pollen and some mold problems, and the region is subjected to periodic cedar burning and spot herbiciding of the state roads, but none of these potential irritants have been major problems for the Pitmans.

The Pitman residence is a beautiful country house that reflects as much on the lifestyle and tastes of its unique owners as it does on the possibilities in healthy housing. It is distinctive for the care with which it is placed in the

Design Team:
Sue Pitman, owner and designer; Mary Oetzel, indoor air quality consultant; Tony Patch, contractor

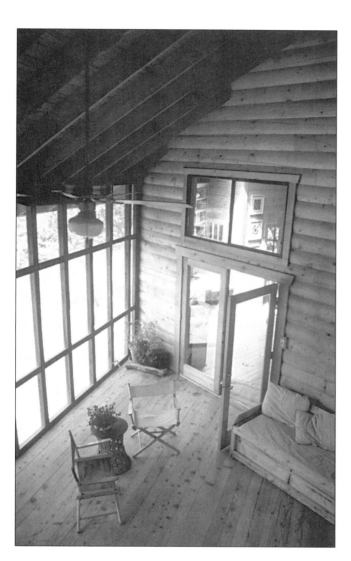

Entrance from the surrounding porch to the "living room" cabin.

landscape and for the open-air lifestyle that its plan supports. It is also notable for the simplicity of its materials and for its innovative architectural approach to coping with the hot and often humid climate.

Both houses are inspired by a traditional southern building form called a "dog run," which is characterized by two log cabin blocks separated by an open breezeway with a common roof and verandah. The first small house is a re-creation of this historical form, while the second version is a larger and more adventurous adaptation of the traditional concept to better suit the family's needs. In both houses the initial idea of a rustic retreat built for the local climate has created homes that are very "healthy by design."

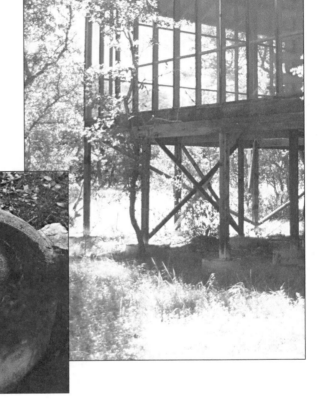

This home stands on posts with specially designed footings to resist insect attack without pesticides (right).

A moat is used to prevent insects from reaching the untreated wood posts (below).

DESIGN PROCESS

Mary Oetzel, a resident of Wimberley and a healthy building consultant, was indirectly involved in the design, as was the contractor. Many of the house's distinctive features were worked out during construction. The ceiling height of the main floor, for example, was raised two feet (60 centimeters) when it became apparent to Sue during construction that its proportions were wrong. This small change gives the house the stately feel and breezy comfort of a southern plantation.

The design of the second house was greatly influenced by the successes and shortcomings of the first. The first house was raised off the ground approximately two feet (60 centimeters) partly to allow inspection of the piers for termites. Inspection proved to be possible but still unpleasant work, and so the second house was raised a full eight feet (2.4 meters) off the ground to make the inspection effortless. The first house had a continuous verandah eight feet wide, which was found slightly too small for real outdoor living. In the second house the cabins were placed at an angle to one another to create the magnificent porch that now defines the character of the house and provides a dramatic center space.

The house is a dramatic example of designing for outdoor living. Nearly half the living area of the house is contained on the porch, and passive ventilation strategies in large measure give the structure its form and ambiance.

Lifting the house off the ground exposes its wooden piers for termite inspection and it allows the house to catch the prevailing breeze without clearing the forest that surrounds it. The house is elongated along its east/west axis with the main entry and porch orientation to the south, facing both the winter sun and the southern summer breeze. The effect of the breeze is amplified by the placement of the two cabins, which together act as wind scoops and direct air through the center of the house. The corners of the cabins touch the northern wall of the porch, creating an opening to the north that can be closed off in the winter with storm windows. With the northern winter winds directed around the house rather than through it, the central area of the porch is habitable year round without additional storm windows.

Within the immense screened enclosure, one log cabin houses only the sleeping rooms while the other houses the living, dining and study areas as well as the kitchen and bath. The plan consolidates the "wet" rooms, the kitchen and single bath, to minimize potential mold problems.

The porch contains most of the house's storage space. In one corner is a cabinet with the teenage son's model airplane supplies, along with the household cleaning supplies. A garment closet opening onto another area of the porch is metal lined to prevent insect infestation and is equipped with its own portable dehumidifier for particularly humid times. Shaker pegs decorate much of the porch's remaining wall space, allowing clothes and other items to be stored before entering the inner houses.

The television is housed on the porch, set up on wheels within casework that allows it to be rolled out of sight when not in use. (Televisions, in particular, can be offensive to a person with multiple chemical sensitivities, because of the amount of plastic and the high temperatures inside the case, which produce fried dust and offgassing from the plastic.) The master bed is also on wheels and is rolled onto the porch most of the year. The bed is rolled back into the bedroom during the day where a dehumidifier can dry the bedding, especially in the damp spring months. In general, Sue appre-

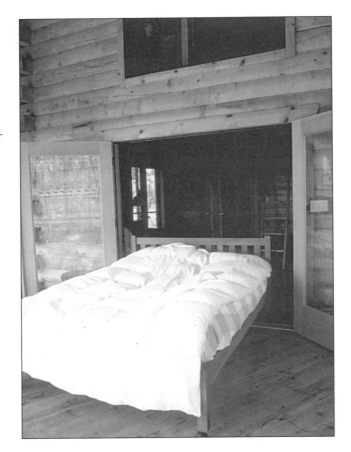

ciates the ability to move from place to place and thus avoid being constantly exposed to the same irritants.

The final key to the health of the home is the detached garage and laundry with a large and carefully isolated storage room above. The detached storage allows the family to separate themselves from most of their belongings without throwing them away, making the process of creating a safe haven less emotionally draining than it often is. As both Sue's and her children's health has gradually improved, family items have one by one been admitted into the main house.

Sue holds residential pesticide responsible for the failure of both her own and her children's health, and so the houses had to use nontoxic pest management strategies to protect both the house and its inhabitants from insects.

Termites and fire ants are major concerns and the design of the posts that lift the house off the ground respond to the problem in several ways. The untreated but easily accessible posts are held by conventional metal seats anchored in concrete footings that protrude above the ground by several inches (10 centimeters). The top of each footing is shaped to form a shallow moat around its post seat. This moat is filled with soapy water during fire ant season; the water stops the ants and the soap prevents mosquitoes from breeding in the shallow pool.

The minimal caulking between logs and the metal lining of the linen closet are both physical barriers to insect infestation. The legs of the beds sit in traditional water-holding castors that likely served as the inspiration for the house's piers. The ritual of keeping the moats filled and inspected implies constant vigilance, which Sue sees as a tradeoff for a house without poisons.

MATERIALS SELECTION

Sue depended on her common sense and a carefully noted diary to discover the sources of her family's sensitivities. Her chiropractor taught her to pay attention to muscle weakness as a sign of adverse reactions to specific materials. Finally, Sue visited as many houses of people with environmental sensitivities as she could in order to familiarize herself with the healthy housing options available. She found, for example, that she objected to the common healthy house materials of concrete and plaster while she could easily tolerate uses of wood objectionable to others with multiple chemical sensitivities. The Pitmans chose to build the house using traditional log walls, which eliminated most questions of insulation and design of wall cavities. This philosophy of simple materials and assembly runs throughout the house. Pesticide-free beetle-kill spruce logs were transported from a mill in Colorado. A minimum amount of acrylic window, door and siding caulking was used to seal the outside spline of the logs from insect migration. In hindsight Sue would have preferred to have used silicone, which now has almost universal acceptance among those with multiple chemical sensitivities. Though the house is sitting in a cedar forest, the use of cut cedar was rejected due to its strong odor.

All exposed electrical wire is contained within metal conduits and there are no plastic fixtures in the house. With each of these choices tradeoffs were made between performance, durability and/or ease of assembly on the one hand and nontoxicity on the other. In the case of the kitchen counter, for example, certain joints have opened up in part because the use of glue was prohibited. Still, the house has a timeless durability that Sue enjoys.

MECHANICAL SYSTEMS

The house has no built-in mechanical ventilation system, partly because the climate doesn't require it and partly because Sue did not want forced air or the potentially moldy ductwork associated with it. Instead, ceiling fans aid natural ventilation inside and on the porch. Winter heating is provided by movable electric space heaters filled with liquid, as well as by the family's willingness to wear additional layers of clothing for the two months or so of cold weather. Two similarly portable dehumidifiers are used in the summer: one in the closet dedicated to good clothes and linen, and the second to dry out the comforter on the master bed.

The design allows for the natural movement of air inside the two story cabins as well as on the porch. The living cabin is treated as a single, interconnected volume to disperse the humidity generated by cooking and bathing. The living/dining space is open above, while the kitchen space is lofted over with a study. To avoid creating a pocket of still air above the sink at the rear of the kitchen, a transfer grille is cut through to the loft above. The kitchen shelves are open to allow for air movement and the range hood provides the only additional mechanical air movement device.

CONSTRUCTION AND SUPERVISION

The builder is a local contractor who was willing to work with Sue on her specific needs. While the process was difficult and construction supervision demanded Sue's full attention, she had great things to say about his common sense and ability to anticipate problems. Typical for the rural economy of central Texas, the house was built with a great deal of inexpensive labor and little or no heavy equipment. Supervision involved such things as asking that smoking be allowed only outside of the house.

Sue was extremely sick during the construction of the first house, and was not able to supervise its construction to her satisfaction. The sanctuary that the first house provided allowed her to supervise the construction of the larger house.

Sue estimates that the construction of the house cost one and a half times the amount of a conventional house in the same region. This figure is difficult to ascribe specifically to the technical requirements of a healthy house, however, since the solution is such an integrated expression of taste, lifestyle preferences, environmental sensitivities and health concerns.

STAR DIAGRAM ASSESSMENT AND CRITIQUE

The house appears to be very successful in providing a safe haven for the Pitman family, doing so in a way that gives them a wonderful place to live and allows them to enjoy the natural beauty of their surroundings.

Climate responsiveness is at the heart of achieving energy efficiency and this house is exceptionally responsive in a climate where cooling is the dominant energy drain. The house is designed for maximum passive modification of the local flows of sun and wind energy. The only problem that compromises the energy efficiency of the design is that, as with so many houses that seek the cleanest possible air, the rural location entails a long daily commute for at least some of the family.

The house was built before resource efficiency as it is understood in this book was an issue of much public concern. The uniqueness of the house makes superficial comparisons difficult; the solid log walls use more lumber than a conventionally framed house but in their relatively raw state they represent little total embodied energy content. The beetle-kill logs are a positive choice from a resource perspective, though the Colorado source required long distance transportation.

As is often the case, the most debatable decision from a resource point of view clearly reflects the priority of health. The massive deck and roof of the house are constructed of redwood in order to be weather and insect resistant without chemical treatments. Sustainable sources of redwood are rare and most is the result of clear-cutting the ancient forests of the Pacific Northwest.

SUMMARY TABLE

For Whom?

New detached home for a family in which the mother and two children are environmentally hypersensitive.

Climate and Site

The climate is the predominantly hot/humid region of the Texas Hill Country. Approximately 1000 ft. (300 meters) elevation. Large lot in a semi-rural area, distant from highways, industry and agriculture.

The Building

New construction, 1986. Three bedrooms, one bath, kitchen, dining/living room, study and porch space. Laundry and storage located in remote garage.

Design Emphasis

Climatic Design—site- and climate-responsive form maximizing passive ventilation in summer, wind shelter and sun penetration in winter.

135

Energy Efficient Design (envelope systems)—walls are solid timber. Floors and ceilings of fully enclosed spaces insulated with unfaced yellow fiberglass batts. Foil-faced vapor barrier in ceiling of fully enclosed roof may provide some radiant barrier benefits depending on installation.

Resource Efficient—effort to use resource efficient materials. A rain barrel is in use to collect water for gardening.

Air Quality Design—carefully designed to eliminate synthetic and volatile materials and to control insect damage without biocides or pesticides. Innovative space planning, passive ventilation, materials selection and integrated pest management. Potentially irritating activities such as television viewing and hobby activities are located on the enclosed but well-ventilated porch.

Design for Isolation of Pollutants—potential pollutants eliminated rather than isolated, when possible. Rigorous zoning to isolate moisture sources within the house and to isolate storage and automobiles from the house.

Design for Light—south-facing clerestories admit winter sun into the house, while the deep porch provides shade year round. The house is set within a scrub forest, which limits distant views and glare to the south. Unlike a cold climate house, shade rather than light is the priority.

Design for Noise Protection—isolated site, dense vegetation. Within the house the open plan and concern for ventilation work against rigorous acoustic separation between activities.

Design for EMF Protection—Sue Pitman was not aware of this issue at the time of construction. Separation of sleeping areas from appliances and in particular the use of the sleeping porch along with the fact that all wiring is contained in metal conduits presumably works toward EMF avoidance.

Design for Low Maintenance—casual philosophy of natural and minimally finished materials avoids much of the need for finish maintenance. The roof form is simple and effective at shedding water and the body of the house is elevated well away from the ground, reducing moisture and insect attack problems. Increased maintenance requirements of natural insect barriers is accepted in order to eliminate toxic alternatives.

Materials Selection

Walls are pesticide-free beetle-kill logs from a mill in Colorado sealed with acrylic sealant. The decking is unfinished redwood.

Foundations—4x4 wood framing bearing on concrete footings elevates the house eight feet (2.4 meters) above grade.

Frame—roof of rafters supported by a ridge beam bearing on log walls and at perimeter by unsheathed screen walls of 2x4 wood studs making up the perimeter of the porch. Floor is joist framed.

Roofing—redwood with a vapor barrier of foil-faced pressed paperboard constructed without formaldehyde-based glues, and insulated with un-faced yellow fiberglass batts.

Exterior Finishes—clear acrylic sealant.

Insulation—unfaced yellow fiberglass batts used to avoid pink color additives and paper binders.

Windows and Doors—the few doors contained in the house were custom built using solid stock.

Interior Finishes—unfinished dressed face of solid spruce log walls. The painter was required to sand off all exposed wood labels rather than use solvents. No cut cedar used.

Floor Coverings—deck floor unfinished 2x6 redwood planking.

Kitchen Cabinets—unfinished solid pine constructed without glue. The kitchen countertop is pine planks, finished with clear acrylic sealer.

Furnishings—organic cotton futons, simple cotton and solid hardwood furniture, cotton shower curtain.

Other—all exposed electrical wiring is encased in metal conduit to encapsulate vinyl sheathing. All electrical outlets are metal rather than plastic.

Heating, Air Conditioning, Air Filtration and Ventilation

Heating, A/C Type—no central heating or A/C systems. Household wiring adequate for the use of portable electric/oil radiant heaters in coldest months and for portable dehumidifiers in the spring. Two dehumidifiers in use: one in good clothes closet and one that is primarily used in the master bedroom to dry out down bedding during the day in humid weather.

Ventilation System Type—passive ventilation maximized through building siting, massing and space planning. Toilet and range hood each have exhaust fans.

Filtration System Type—well with potassium permanganate iron removal unit and water softener. Reverse osmosis and carbon filtration used for drinking water only.

Other—all appliances are electric due to personal sensitivity to natural gas. The garage houses a washer and dryer, but in keeping with the desire to use natural ventilation over mechanical, clothes are primarily dried on the line outside.

New Low-income Apartment Building for People with Multiple Chemical Sensitivities

STANDARD
PRACTICE

Design Team:
  Kodama and
  Associates,
  Architects (Steve
  Kodama, Principal
  in Charge;
  Kenneth Bishop,
  Project Architect)
Builder:
Joseph DiGiorgio and
  Sons
Developer and Owner:
  Ecology House
  Inc. (Jon
  Marchant,
  President of the
  Board; Katherine
  Crecelius,
  Development
  Consultant)

Name: Ecology House

Location: San Rafael, California, temperate, dry

Ecology House is the first HUD (Housing and Urban Development) funded apartment building designed, constructed and maintained for people with extreme environmental hypersensitivities. A ground-breaking project, Ecology House has attracted a great deal of controversy since opening, but is proving to be a successful step toward healthy, low-income housing. The 11 apartment units are occupied, and although three of the original tenants found the air quality unacceptable and moved out, other tenants report that their health has substantially improved since moving in.

The board and the architects searched for two years before settling on the location for Ecology House. They wanted a rural site, away from potential sources of air pollution, which was difficult to find given the local zoning laws and economic constraints. The final site represents a compromise. The site is on a parcel of land that had been set aside for low-income housing within a larger residential development. The entire development is built on reclaimed marshland adjacent to San Francisco Bay, which provides the cleanest possible air within an otherwise urban area.

DESIGN PROCESS

Ecology House presented a formidable design challenge—creating an acceptable environment for future clients, each with unknown specific health requirements. To meet this challenge, the board of Ecology House Inc. assembled a group of chemically sensitive advisors who volunteered to provide input on design and to screen potential construction materials. The architects were selected based on their long and successful track record of designing nonprofit and special needs housing in the San Fran-

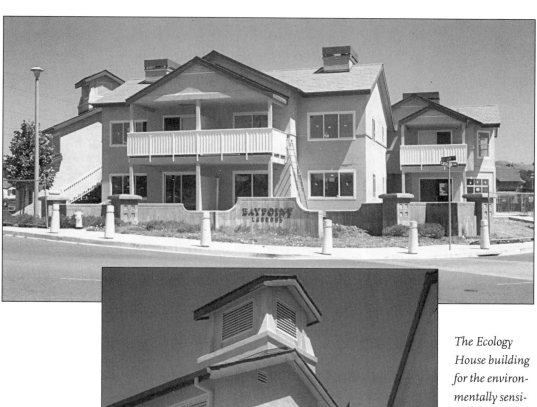

The Ecology House building for the environmentally sensitive (above).

Street gate. The project is integrated into the neighborhood, yet maintains the separation necessary for the environmentally sensitive to control their surroundings (left).

139

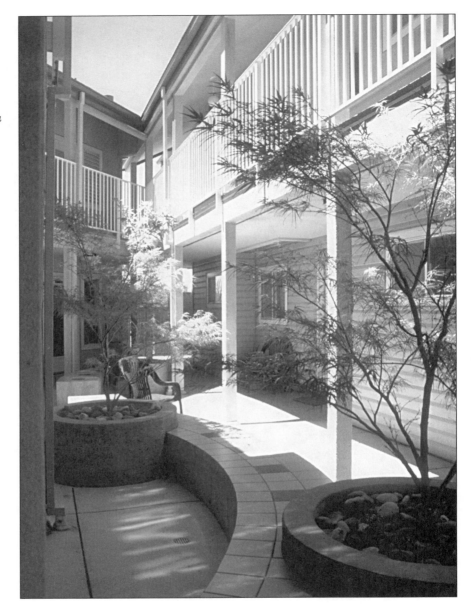

The courtyard provides individual outside entrances for each unit and a sheltered and semi-public space.

cisco area. The general contractors were brought on board early in the process and selected without a bidding process in order to have them participate in the development of the design. Their early involvement was crucial to the success of the project, which depended on the general contractors working with the architect to solve the project's unique problems, and educating the subcontractors about the special health-related requirements of the job.

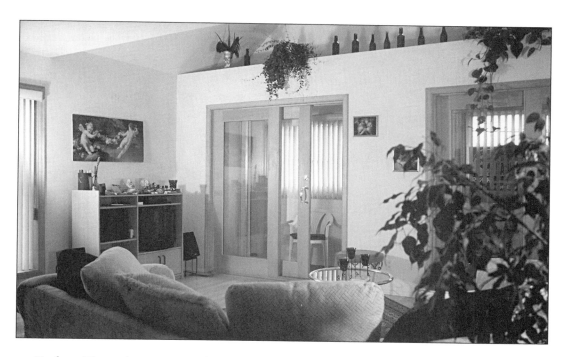

Ecology House is a two-story building housing 11 apartments, which are grouped around a central courtyard and connected by exterior walks. The courtyard scheme was chosen to facilitate passive ventilation, and each unit has operable windows on two sides as well as in each kitchen and bath. An alternative approach would have been to seal the building to allow filtering of the supply air. But the site has a steady breeze, and there was concern over the maintenance of filters in a closed system so an open building was chosen. The open plan was ultimately less expensive.

An elevator makes each unit accessible to the disabled. The elevator, and the building's trash and recycling room, are housed in a separate building from the apartments, guaranteeing isolation of equipment odors and noise. The separate structure also houses an open-air community storage room which allows residents to air out personal belongings before bringing them into their units.

The units are designed for accessibility, and have generous passage dimensions. At the same time, they make the most of their limited size. For example, the coat closets at each front door are metal units which can be moved to make room for a wheelchair-bound occupant.

A great deal of attention was devoted to minimizing the electromagnetic fields. In the kitchen the refrigerators and electric stoves are set against the outside wall rather than the wall between units to ensure that their fields aren't directed toward habitable space.

This interior has been personalized with carefully chosen elements, based on individual acceptability. The result is rich and welcoming.

MATERIALS SELECTION

The choice of materials for Ecology House sets it apart from a conventional project. Like many healthy housing projects, it avoids asphalt, formaldehyde-emitting materials, pressure-treated wood, finishes that require on-site painting or gluing, carpeting and finishes which could trap odors and dust.

Long-term durability was another important issue, because even routine maintenance was likely to expose the residents to unacceptable irritants. The desire for both irritant- and maintenance-free materials conflicted with the financial constraints of the project, and the need for manufacturer's warranties. These often disallow substitute materials that would eliminate offensive components, and warranties may require specific materials such as sealers, which may not be acceptable to the sensitive.

The project was framed with wood rather than metal studs for cost reasons and insulated with fiberglass batts. The walls, including uninsulated interior partitions, were encapsulated with aluminum foil to ensure that insulation and wood odors would not contaminate the living spaces. Some plywood sheathing containing glue was used in the exterior walls to meet California earthquake codes, but all of the interior shear walls and subfloors use traditional diagonal wood bracing and planking.

Conventional gypsum wall board was eliminated due to the unpredictability of the facing paper's chemical content. Painted wall surfaces were ruled out because repainting for each new tenant could cause adverse reactions among others in the building, even if the paint would be acceptable when dry. The eventual choice was a veneer plaster system applied to a gypsum backer board.

The one potentially compromising material is the fire sprinkler piping, which is PVC pipe assembled with PVC glue, but various precautions seem to have prevented any problems. All of the exposed components of the system are metal and the plastic is isolated from the living space by each apartment's continuous foil lining. Most of the piping is in the attic, which is fan ventilated, and all of it was installed long before occupancy to allow the solvents in the glue to offgas.

The courtyard is the centerpiece of Ecology House. The use of resinous trees or pollen-producing plants was out of the question due to the sensitivities of the occupants, and planting was further constrained by local water conservation ordinances. The result is a patterned hard surface courtyard with planters that are sculpturally interesting in themselves, containing only low-pollen, naturally pest- and drought-resistant plants. Irrigation is provided by a buried drip system.

MECHANICAL SYSTEMS

Although individual gas-fired forced air furnaces are typical for low-cost housing in California, Ecology House uses a central gas-fired boiler to supply hot water to baseboard convectors. This eliminates natural gas odors and the potential for contaminated ductwork in individual units.

The kitchens and baths are mechanically vented to the roof, with the fans mounted far enough away to allow acoustical and electrical field isolation. Fans also vent all attic spaces to cool the building and prevent odors from sun-baked roofing and insulation from entering the units.

The project conforms to California energy codes, except for the substitution of incandescent for fluorescent lighting.

CONSTRUCTION AND SUPERVISION

The job site was kept very clean, and regular meetings were held with subcontractors to explain the health-related goals of the job. Careful precautions were taken to avoid introducing potential contaminants to the job site. Smoking was not allowed on the site. Paint spray cans, often used for marking rough construction, were not allowed. Only nontoxic cleaners were used during and after construction. Workers were asked to park away from the building, and even concrete trucks were kept at a distance when delivering their loads. The limited amount of plywood that was used in the building was stored offsite so it could air before being installed.

STAR DIAGRAM ASSESSMENT AND CRITIQUE

While 3 of the original 11 tenants were unable to tolerate the newly completed units and the resulting publicity was extremely negative, Ecology House is now fully occupied and the board feels increasingly justified in calling it a success. As noted, several current residents report that their health has substantially improved due to the safe haven that the building provides. Ecology House cost approximately 11% more than conventional HUD funded housing for this site, or approximately $18,000 US extra per unit in a $1.8 million project. Most of this money was for material substitutions.

The natural ventilation has worked well, as have most of the material choices, though the use of additive-free concrete has resulted in minor cracking. The use of the veneer plaster system has had mixed results, with half of the residents in favor of it and half not tolerating it well. The walls

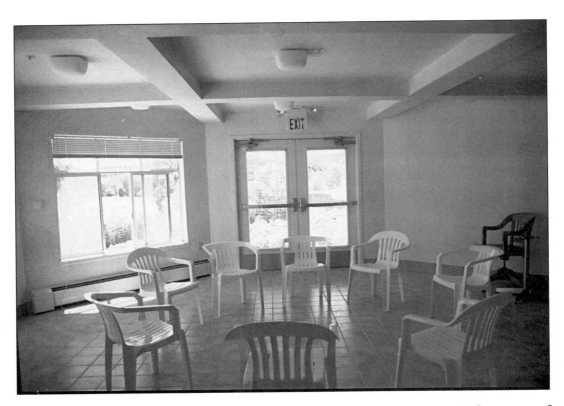

A meeting room in the common area is designed to be acceptable to all occupants.

and ceiling of one unit have subsequently been sealed with four coats of nontoxic acrylic sealer on a trial basis. The tile floors are appreciated by all residents, but the grout was left unsealed and now tends to rub loose, creating a minor annoyance. The baked-enamel kitchen cabinets have proven to be the most contentious item, peeling and producing complaints about odors. No one is certain about the source of odors or why the cabinets are deteriorating. Ecology House Inc. would now recommend stainless-steel cabinets.

The whole house water filtration system is a success, though the carbon filter is somewhat expensive to keep charged.

SUMMARY TABLE

For Whom?

A range of environmentally hypersensitive occupants

Climate and Site

Mild Mediterranean-like coastal climate. The site is on San Francisco Bay in San Rafael, California.

The Building

Eleven units of low-income housing for people with multiple chemical sensitivities.

Design Emphasis

Climatic Design—courtyard plan for optimal passive ventilation.

Energy Efficient Design (envelope systems)—envelope meets California Energy Code Requirements.

Resource Efficient Design—deemed a conflict because the use of recycled-content materials might introduce added chemicals.

Air Quality Design—cross-ventilation of all units. Community open-air storage room for initial airing out. Private balconies with privacy screens accommodating exterior storage of personal belongings. Extreme care in materials selection to eliminate sources of potential contamination and facilitate house cleaning.

Design for Isolation of Pollutants—elevator and trash/recycling room completely isolated. All wood framing isolated from the interior by foil encapsulation.

Design for Light—all units are well daylit.

Design for Noise Protection—elevator and trash/recycling room physically removed from apartments. Kitchen and bath exhaust fans isolated.

Design for EMF Protection—Ecology House sits near high-voltage lines that make it unworkable for people with high EMF sensitivities. The power lines were tested and their fields were found to be within generally acceptable limits. Within the project, no fluorescent lighting is used; appliances are located on exterior rather than common walls; interior wiring is aluminum cable; power to individual units is distributed through the attic rather than walls, metal shielding is used to isolate the transformer, electrical switch boxes and exhaust fans; and power lines to the elevator mechanical room are buried underground in continuous rigid conduit.

Design for Low Maintenance—fiber cement shingle roof and colored cement stucco/metal siding exterior walls will require no repainting. A shop-painted metal roof was desired for lowest possible maintenance but rejected on the basis of cost. Additional funds were raised to substitute powder-coated aluminum for wood exterior trellises, fences and gates.

Materials Selection

Foundations—additive-free concrete slab on grade thermally isolated by rigid polystyrene foamboard to prevent moisture problems. The project is built on structural fill.

Frame—standard wood stud construction. Diagonal bracing and diagonal plank flooring used except where earthquake codes required plywood as exterior sheathing.

Roofing—fiber cement shingles on plywood roof sheathing and asphalt-saturated roofing felt. The manufacturer's 50-year guarantee on the shingles required the use of the asphalt underlay or an alternative would have been used.

Exterior Finishes—steel siding with factory-baked enamel paint and cement plaster stucco with integral color. Aluminum trim was fabricated for miscellaneous trim and powder-coat painted offsite. Roof fascia, downspouts and watertable trim were fabricated on site from galvanized sheet metal and painted with low-odor paint.

Insulation—fiberglass batt insulation and aluminum foil vapor barrier.

Windows and Doors—double-glazed, aluminum frame, sliding windows and patio doors. Aluminum mini-blinds with baked-enamel finish. Steel exterior and interior doors. Insulated doors use foamboard insulation. Doors factory primed and painted off site with fast drying automobile paint. Frames factory-baked polyester paint. Bifold closet doors steel with baked-enamel finish.

Interior Finishes—two-coat veneer plaster system, unfinished. Three-coat plaster on cement board in baths. Shower tile set in thickset mortar bed.

Floor Coverings—glazed quarry tile set in a full bed of additive-free cement mortar. Cement grout with sand, unsealed.

Kitchen Cabinets—steel with baked-enamel finish.

Other—countertops of stainless steel, all electrical fixtures ceramic, all plumbing either cast iron or copper.

Heating, Air Conditioning, Air Filtration and Ventilation

Heating, A/C Type—centrally located and remotely vented gas-fired boiler supplying hydronic baseboard convectors. No A/C provided.

Ventilation System Type—passive ventilation supplemented by exhaust fans for kitchens and baths. Fans mounted remotely to isolate electromagnetic fields, noise, and motor offgassing. Attic spaces similarly vented by fan to prevent contaminant buildup and aid cooling.

Filtration System Type—no air filtration provided.

Other—whole house water filtration system supplies all domestic water, including water used for showers and toilets.

CHAPTER 8

Systems

HEATING AND AIR CONDITIONING

Passive Solar Heating

Passive solar heating is appropriate for most climates in North America, except those that receive little sunlight in winter. Passive solar means that sunlight is used and stored directly, without the use of special collectors, liquids, pumps, pipes and ducts. Solar design usually requires south- and east-facing windows located so that the sun will directly heat the home in winter. Shading must be provided to prevent too much sunlight from entering in the summer. In a conventional home, in a moderate climate, solar heat can account for about 10% of the home's annual heating requirements without extraordinary efforts. With careful design, extra insulation, high-performance windows and massive walls and floors to store heat, solar heat can contribute 40% or more. By extraordinary efforts, this amount can be raised to 80%, even in a cold, northerly climate. In the southwest, where there is a lot of winter sun, solar can easily contribute over 60% of heating needs. With some extra effort, it can provide 90% of heating needs.

Passive solar is an ideal heating method for the healthy home. It provides sunlit interiors in winter, can perform without fans and ducts, does not stir up dust, and uses the only truly environmentally sustainable energy source. Designing a passive solar home is more critical, however, than if solar control is not optimized. Positioning windows, choosing insulation levels, locating concrete or other massive materials to store heat, and designing shading for summer must all be carefully considered. It is best to consult an energy expert, and use a computer simulation tool to optimize solar features.

Forced-Air Heating

A forced-air system has a heating or cooling unit which recirculates house air. The basic components are a fan, a burner (or another heat source such as a hot water coil) an optional air conditioning coil, filters and ductwork.

Though a forced-air system can be an appropriate choice for healthy housing, not all forced-air heating systems are alike.

Most furnaces burn natural gas, propane, fuel oil or wood right inside the unit, or they may have an electric coil. These are *not* preferred for healthy housing. An alternative type of furnace does not contain a burner, but receives heating or cooling from a remote boiler or heat pump/air conditioning compressor. This type is called a fan coil. A fan coil has significant advantages for healthy housing because the heat exchange temperature is lower. Heat exchangers which maintain temperatures below about 180°F (85°C) do not tend to cook dust and produce "burnt odors" the way high-temperature units, such as those with gas or oil burners or electric coils do. Also, with a fan coil, any fuel burner providing the hot water to the coil can be isolated from the home to prevent flue gas from entering. See the Heating and Ventilating section of the 79 Best Healthy Building Solutions.

The fan-coil furnace can also be supplied by a heat pump. Heat pumps are variants of refrigeration units which are primarily designed for heating homes. They normally function to heat the home, providing heat extracted from outdoor air or the earth, but they can be set up to cool also. Heating with a heat pump has several advantages for the healthy home, especially where electricity is the main fuel available. Heat pump coils stay below 180°F (85°C) so they are not likely to cook dust. They use less than half the electricity required for conventional electric heat, and in cooling mode they will dehumidify to maintain comfortable, healthy conditions in humid climates. Unfortunately, they are expensive to buy and install. However, if cooling is needed and electricity will be used for heating, they may be a good investment. Your utility company or an energy consultant can do a cost and payback analysis for you.

Fan-coil forced-air systems are generally healthier than electric baseboard heaters, or conventional gas, oil and electric furnaces, but all have the problem of dust accumulation when dust falls on the heat exchanger. Fortunately, filters help to reduce the problem by trapping dust before it reaches the hot surface. Forced-air systems can also easily incorporate ventilation to all rooms. Probably the healthiest forced-air system is a hot water or heat pump furnace with a continuous fan, and high-performance filtration. This unit has a low-temperature coil, reducing the hot dust problem, and the fans are usually strong enough to work with a good filter. A system heated by a separate boiler can also provide air conditioning with the addition of a cooling coil and compressor/condenser. A system supplied by a heat pump can provide cooling by reversing the heating cycle. Duct design is also an important factor in healthy forced-air systems.

A fan-coil furnace has numerous advantages for the healthy home.

148

Convection Heating Systems

These systems rely on the buoyancy of heated air as it passes over a warm coil or tube. The heated air rises up the wall, and cooler air flows in from below to be warmed. The heaters are usually long, thin, baseboard-mounted units. They may use electricity, or be supplied with hot water circulated from an electric- or fuel-fired central boiler. Systems using circulated hot water are sometimes called hydronic. There are also "cabinet convectors" which are mounted in a box in the wall or floor, which may have a small fan to assist air circulation.

Conventional electric baseboard heat is usually the worst system for indoor air quality for four reasons:

- It has no means of drawing air into the home or exhausting it the way a forced-air system has, and so ventilation must be provided separately.
- The surfaces of the coils collect dust which then is vaporized and carbonized when the heat is on. This explains the characteristic "hot dust" odors, especially when the heat is first turned on in the fall.
- Electric heat is expensive, and because each room has an individual thermostat, people tend to shut off unused rooms in winter, causing moisture damage. No room should be set below 60°F (15°C) during the heating season.
- There is no filtration to control dust.

If electric baseboard heaters are the chosen heating method, it is best to use a sealed, liquid-filled type. These are somewhat larger than a conventional electric heater with the same heat output, but they use the same electrical connections, and allow easy individual control of rooms by local thermostats. Portable, liquid-filled electric units are also available, and are a good solution for heating an individual room without having to modify the wiring (if the existing wiring is adequate). See the Heating section in 79 Best Healthy Building Solutions for illustrations. Special heaters with all-stainless-steel parts are also available for those who may be sensitive to painted heater parts.

Though convection heating has merit, since it cannot provide ventilation a separate air distribution system must be installed for ventilation, filtration or air conditioning in hot or cold climates. For a healthy house in a cold climate using convection heat, a fully ducted ventilation system is recommended, similar to the one shown in the Heating and Ventilating section in 79 Best Healthy Building Solutions.

Radiant Heating Systems

Radiant heating systems function by heating people and objects directly, rather than heating the air in the room. We all experience radiant heating when we are outside on a cold sunny day, and can feel the warmth of the sun. Conversely, a room with a large cold window will feel cold, even if the room air temperature is comfortable. This is because the body loses radiant heat to the cold glass.

Radiant home heating requires heating large surfaces such as floors, walls and ceilings, or it can be done with large metal radiators in each room (like the old steam systems). Massive central heaters made of brick and tile in the European tradition are also sometimes used in healthy homes. Radiant heated floors have important advantages because human comfort is regulated, to a large extent, by the temperature of the feet. In winter, having your feet just slightly above the temperature of your head will help you to feel comfortable, even with moderately cool air temperatures, though this is a matter of preference. In summer, a massive, cool floor will help you to feel cooler. Heated floors and ceilings typically operate at about 75° to 80°F (24° to 27°C). Radiant floors or ceilings provide uniform comfort with minimal air currents, and without the side effects, such as dust stirring and odors from heated dust associated with high-temperature systems. Remember that radiant heated ceilings will also heat the floor above, and concrete slab floors with radiant heating on ground level will require perimeter and subslab insulation to reduce heat loss to the soil. For concrete slab construction in a moderate or cold climate, radiant floor heating is preferred by many people for comfort.

Radiant heating is mostly done with a hot water source circulating water through tubes buried in floors. Rooms can be individually zoned using electric valves which are connected to thermostats. The thermostat should *not* be a conventional wall type which measures air temperature. It should have a probe buried in the heated surface to measure the actual surface temperature. Ceilings can be heated with a hot water tube system buried in plaster, but this is relatively rare and expensive. Most ceiling radiant heating is done with electric cables set in gypsum panels, but this system is not often used in healthy houses due to concerns about electromagnetic field exposures.

Like low-temperature convection heating, radiant heating has merit for a healthy home, but it cannot provide ventilation, filtration or air conditioning. A separate air distribution system must be installed for these purposes. For a healthy house using radiant heat in a cold climate, a fully ducted ventilation system is recommended, similar to the one shown in the Heating section of 79 Best Healthy Building Solutions.

A separate ventilation and possibly filtration system may be necessary with radiant or convective heating, but it is still a preferred heating type.

Wood Heating

Wood heating is common in suburban and rural areas today, particularly in cold and moderate climate zones. Though wood is a renewable fuel, most wood-burning appliances are very inefficient, and produce substantial air pollution. The problem is so serious in some colder regions that severe restrictions on burning are applied to reduce "winter smog."

If a woodburning heater is to be used in a healthy home, there are some healthy and efficient choices available. A massive heater, such as a European "tile oven," can be used to burn wood rapidly and efficiently, because it stores the heat for many hours afterward. It does not need to have the air restricted to control it, the way a lightweight steel stove does, causing a smoky fire. If a tile oven is not possible, then a good EPA-listed woodburning stove with a catalytic burner is another option. These burn cleanly, as long as the wood is dry and the air control is not fully closed. Another option is the pellet stove. These burn manufactured wood pellets made from sawmill waste. They are very efficient and clean burning compared to other wood stoves. All woodburners tend to release some soot, smoke and ash into the home. They also may have high surface temperatures causing carbonized dust.

Furnace Fans

The furnace fan is important to successful air filtration and comfort. Older furnaces generally have clumsy, belt-driven fans which are not very effective at pulling air through a good filter. They only operate when the furnace is on, and are likely to be noisy. A good furnace fan now has an integral motor, is quiet, capable of pulling air through a very restrictive filter, and operates on low speed most of the time. The fan only switches to high speed when needed for heating or cooling. This is called "continuous fan operation." The advantage of continuous operation is that the air is constantly filtered, ventilation is assured, and air is prevented from "stratifying," that is, the warm and cool air stay mixed instead of the warmer air all rising to the ceiling. A good furnace fan also uses 40% less electricity than its predecessor did two decades ago. The most efficient type are called "electronically controlled motors."

Furnace Venting

Any type of combustion unit in the home must be reliably vented to prevent dangerous flue gases from entering. In a healthy home, every boiler, furnace or water heater which burns fuel should be a "sealed combustion" type (see the Heating section in 79 Healthy Building Solutions), or located in a furnace room with a chimney which is separate from the dwelling space. A sealed combustion burner is fully enclosed, and connected by sealed pipes to an outside air supply and a combustion gas vent. Older types of burners which are not vented this way should be replaced, or isolated from the dwelling, when major renovations are being done. This is especially important to prevent chimney backdrafting.

Air Conditioning

Residential air conditioners are electric, motor-driven refrigeration units with cooling coils, mounted either in a central furnace, or in a smaller, room-sized unit. They discharge heat either to outdoor air, or to the earth. In warm climates, air conditioning provides comfort when outdoor air is too warm, humid or polluted to be used for cooling. It can be a useful part of a healthy building strategy because it dehumidifies the building's interior, and provides cooling of recirculated air and filtered indoor air. Because cooling air reduces its capacity to hold moisture, a cooling unit will also remove moisture from indoor air. This moisture will accumulate as condensate on the evaporation coils in the home, and must be collected and sent to a drain. Trapped moisture in cooling equipment is a serious health risk because it is easily contaminated by bacteria and fungi. Maintaining clean cooling coils and keeping condensate drains clear is absolutely essential in the healthy home. Ventilation may also be drastically reduced during cooling periods, which also contributes to unhealthy conditions.

Air conditioning uses a lot of energy, and may be noisy. Building design should be optimized to minimize equipment needs, and equipment should be installed to minimize noise. Outside compressors should be located away from neighbors and bedrooms, and should be screened with dense landscaping and fences to absorb noise.

Small local air conditioners are also available, called "split units," which can be used for a single room. These are far better quality than the window-mounted type of room air conditioner.

In very hot, dry regions, another type of air conditioner is available called an evaporative system or "swamp cooler." These use a moistened, fabric-covered heat exchanger with a small fan. Evaporation extracts heat from the indoor air stream or heat exchange liquid as it passes through. These provide safe and environmentally appropriate cooling in dry regions, however, the water source and evaporator must be kept clean to prevent fungal and bacterial contamination.

A massive wood-fired heater can be appropriate for the healthy home if it is a clean burning design.

HUMIDIFICATION

Humidification is important in colder regions where winter dryness is a problem, particularly for people with respiratory difficulties. One humidification method uses a humidifier on a forced-air system which passes part of the air stream through an absorbent material moistened with a water spray. A humidity control can be used to turn the system on automatically when needed. Unfortunately, this type of humidifier is prone to biological growth, because it holds water at room temperature, and can accumulate dust and debris which will support bacteria and fungi.

If humidification of a forced-air system is important for health reasons, and a "wick" and "drum" type unit is used, careful cleaning and maintenance are essential. The water supply should be fresh, directly from the pipe, and not held in a reservoir for long periods. The wick or drum should be washed with a mild vinegar solution at least every three months, and replaced when it becomes soiled. Electronic, "ultrasonic" humidifiers are available which do not use wicks or drums but vaporize the water directly. These are more costly, but safer to operate. Hot steam units are also available, but these use a lot of electricity. If the home has no forced-air system, the old method of placing pans of water on warm surfaces can be used in winter.

VENTILATION

Ventilation is the extraction of stale air from indoors, and the introduction of outdoor air to replace it. Ventilation may be provided by openings in the building which encourage air movement and catch breezes, or it may be provided by fans when the building is closed up. High ventilation rates also aid cooling when outdoor air is not too hot. Ventilation is also, among other things, a moisture control issue. Every bath and laundry should have a quiet and effective exhaust fan, and it should be used regularly for odor and moisture control. In the kitchen, be sure to have an effective range hood which is ducted to the outdoors. The quieter it is, the more likely it is to be used regularly. If you have a forced-air furnace, be sure it has a combustion air intake duct (required by gas code in most areas) because this will help to provide outdoor air in the home when the exhaust fans are used.

If you want the best ventilation system for a cold climate, consider a continuous, balanced system such as a heat recovery ventilator (HRV). These can be ducted through a furnace, or to the rooms by a separate, small-diameter duct system. (See the Ventilating section in 79 Healthy Building Solutions) They usually take the place of the bath and laundry exhaust fans. The outside air intake to an HRV can be carefully located and filtered to provide the best available air supply, avoiding local sources of pollens, dust, auto exhaust, and so on. Retrofitting an HRV to an existing home can be difficult, however. Consult a ventilation expert, and if you have an older home, be prepared to make substantial improvements to draft sealing so that the system will work properly.

You should also be aware that adding a high-capacity exhaust, such as a downdraft cooktop or grill in the kitchen, can cause conventional gas flues and fireplaces to backdraft, introducing dangerous gases, smoke and soot. This is another good reason to consult a ventilation expert.

In a very mild climate, ventilation is usually provided by opening windows for most of the year, providing that the outdoor air quality is adequate. Even in a severe climate, opening windows can provide ventilation and cooling for a few months. If outdoor air quality is very poor, then a ventilation and filtration system is advisable.

Forced-Air Ductwork

Humidity control is usually very important in the healthy home.

The design of forced-air ductwork is very important. It determines how effective heating, cooling and ventilation will be, how easily the system can be kept clean and how much noise it will make. In the healthy home, all of the ducts should be accessible for cleaning, and designed to avoid trapping dust and debris. In healthy homes it is important to use only fully sheet-metal-lined ducts and to wash new ductwork with a mild washing soda solution to remove oily debris left from manufacturing. Washing the ducts prevents odors from residue, and the capture of dust by sticky duct surfaces. Return ducts (those which bring air back to the furnace or air conditioner) should *not* be built using wood joists or wall studs as part of the duct, though it is allowed by code in some areas (see the Heating and Ventilating section in 79 Best Healthy Building Solutions).

Also, do not use any form of duct liner which may trap dust or release fiber or adhesive odors. Duct liners are fiberglass panels sometimes used in heating and air conditioning systems, to reduce equipment noise and to control sound transfer between rooms through the ductwork. Equipment noise can be isolated from the ducts by using a short, flexible duct connector made of heat-resistant fabric. Mylar-coated foil, or aluminum accordion duct can be used if the fabric is unacceptable to the sensitive individual. Sizing ducts properly will help to reduce the "velocity noise" or whistle problem at the grilles. Noise transfer between rooms served by the same system is more difficult to control. Individual ducts run back to the furnace, instead of branched ducts to adjacent rooms, will help in these situations.

154

Both heating and air conditioning ducts should always be located inside the building insulation to reduce the risk of condensation collecting in the duct. Where this is not possible, the duct should be fitted with an outside insulation sleeve, securely covered, and sealed with aluminum foil. All ducts should be sealed at every joint to reduce loss of air and to limit outside contamination. Metal foil tape is the preferred sealing method for the healthy home. Cloth, plastic tape or liquid sealers containing solvents are not appropriate.

Integrating Ventilation With a Forced-Air System

Forced-air systems can be easily adapted to provide ventilation for the healthy home, because they have ducts connected to each room. Adaptation is done simply by introducing an outside air intake to the return duct of the furnace, just before the filters. The fan will tend to draw air in from outside, mix it with recirculated air, then deliver it to the rooms. This air should then be exhausted by a fan (or fans) extracting air from the kitchen, washrooms and laundry, where odors and moisture are generated. In the healthy home, air is also sometimes extracted from the closets or storage areas in order to prevent odors from contaminated items from entering the home. For example, clothing which has been worn around smokers or exposed to mothballs will release odors which are objectionable to sensitive people. These can be isolated in a closet with an exhaust.

In cold regions, intake air must be preheated before it enters the furnace, to avoid comfort problems and equipment failure. The best way to preheat intake air is to extract heat from the exhaust air, using a heat recovery ventilator, or exhaust heat pump unit. These devices take heat from the outgoing air and transfer it to the intake air. They may add $1,000 US or more to the cost of a system, but they pay for themselves in heating cost savings in cold climates. In a mild region, air can simply be introduced into the furnace return without preheating. The inlet should be located so that is unlikely to draw in auto exhaust, combustion exhaust, dryer exhaust, odors from bathrooms, or kitchen exhaust, and pollen and dust. This is usually done by keeping it well above the ground, and at least several feet away from other vents and plant materials. Locating the intake under the roof soffit is often a good choice. See the Heating and Ventilation section in 79 Best Healthy Building Solutions for illustrations.

Forced-air systems are not for everyone, and they are intentionally avoided in some healthy buildings. They have disadvantages which make them unacceptable for some people, and incompatible with some designs. For example, they produce constant air movement, and some noise. Moving air also tends to dry the skin more than still air, which is a problem for those with dry skin. Also, if dust is introduced into the building, or stirred up by cleaning, it will be blown around until the filters can trap it. Some people feel that air which is recirculated through ducts is less fresh, no matter how clean the system. This may be due, in part, to the tendency for ions (electrically charged molecules) to be lost in ducts, and some people feel invigorated by ions.

Another significant design reason for avoiding forced air is that it mixes all of the air in the building together, which makes zoning, or separating, of individual rooms for air quality reasons virtually impossible. For example, if someone in the household is very sensitive to cooking odors, or if someone has hobbies or personal habits which conflict with the clean air needs of another, the odors cannot be contained if they are served by the same forced-air system. Some of the healthy building examples in this book illustrate how a building has been "zoned" to keep unavoidable air pollutants in one location away from another. This is usually done by using radiant or convector heat, and possibly localized air conditioning, or filtration, instead of a central system which mixes all the air together. Of course, if the entire building is kept to the same standards required by the most sensitive occupant, zoning is not necessary and a forced-air system may be appropriate.

Kitchen Exhaust

Every kitchen needs a quiet, effective exhaust unit above the stove to remove odors, carbon monoxide, nitrogen oxides and excess moisture from cooking. It must be discharged to outside. Beware of kitchen range hoods which only recirculate air through a filter. They are not effective.

The most effective systems are those with a hood mounted above the range which is enclosed by a wall at the back, and ideally by a wall on both sides of the range. The unit should have at least a 200 cfm (cubic feet per minute) capacity on high speed. Those with a remote mounted blower are quieter than those with the blower built into the hood, and centrifugal (squirrel cage) fans are much quieter and more effective than propeller fans. A downdraft range exhaust, such as the type used with countertop grilles, is far less effective than a hood because it must pull air horizontally past pots and pans. It will need at least 500 cfm maximum capacity to work adequately.

Central Vacuums

A built-in vacuum can be an important part of a healthy home. Conventional portable vacuums release a great deal of dust while in use, partly due

Duct design and integration of ventilation is essential to a successful forced-air system.

to the inability of the filter bag to contain fine particles, and partly due to the disturbance of dust by the air which is blown out of the unit. Furthermore, the motors in vacuums commonly produce ozone and oily odors when operated. A built-in vacuum is very effective because the motor is large, and the dust storage is remote from the user. Motorized cleaning heads are also available, for some models, which are driven by air pressure and do not contain electrical motors.

Ideally, the motor and dust storage unit should be outside the occupied areas of the home, and the motor exhaust should be ducted outdoors. This way the dust bag is not cleaned in the home, and the dust and odors in the exhaust are sent outside. In an existing house or apartment where a built-in vacuum is difficult to install, or where cost is prohibitive, there are high-performance portable vacuums available which have some of the advantages of built-in systems. These may use very high-performance (HEPA standard) filters to minimize the fine dust released by their use. They are sometimes called "allergy vacuums."

AIR FILTERS

Air filters must be a part of any forced-air heating or cooling system, or any ventilation system in the healthy home. Filters are also used in recirculating air cleaners which may be portable or built in. Most filters are designed only to remove particles such as house dust, soot and pollens from the air stream; however, special filters will also remove gases such as cooking odors, and unavoidable volatile pollutants.

Particle filters are divided into efficiency types, indicating how well they trap small dust particles. Odor filters are classified by the type of gases they will trap.

Basically, all types of filters may be used in forced-air systems, ventilation systems, or special air-cleaning systems. The critical factors are to have the right filter type for the air pollutants present, and to have the correct size, configuration and fan capacity for the system.

In a typical forced-air system a good deal of fine dust gets drawn into the return air inlets and some travels past the filter. Some of this lands on the heat exchanger,which becomes very hot when the burner is on. The heated dust has a strong odor (that smell when the furnace burner first comes on in the fall) and most of it will turn into fine soot which will be blown into the house. That is why the furnace filter is such a key component in dust control. Filter efficiency is an important factor in forced-air systems. All filters will capture some of the largest dust particles which are visible in bright

157

light, or as dust collected on surfaces. However, these particles are not easily inhaled, and are therefore more of a housekeeping nuisance than a health risk. Small particles, less than 10 microns (ten-thousandths of a millimeter) in diameter are invisible, and easily inhaled deep into the bronchia and lungs, where they may incite allergic reactions or aggravate health problems. Most pollens, mold spores and some fine soot from combustion are less than 10 microns. This fine dust is also the most capable of remaining airborne, so a forced system without efficient filters is certain to be recirculating inhalable dust throughout the home.

Fabric Filters

Your basic furnace filter (the kind you can buy on sale for $1.49) is a crude sieve, capable of preventing furniture, pets, loose books and other large objects from being drawn into the furnace. It will also stop large fibers and clumps of dust. But it doesn't do much for the fine dust that is the most easily inhaled. Ironically, these filters actually work fairly well when they are almost completely clogged, but by then the airflow through them is so sluggish that your furnace may not work properly. This type of filter should be left on the shelf at your bargain store, not put into your furnace.

Pleated fabric filters are the most common, medium-efficiency replace-

The right kitchen exhaust and vacuum are also important parts of the healthy home.

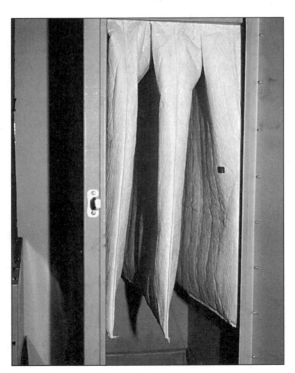

A polyester fabric bag type filter installed in a fan-coil furnace, 80% efficient by the Atmospheric Method.

ments for standard furnace filters. They are several times more efficient than conventional filters. These are from one to four inches (2.5 to 10 cm) thick, and contain a pleated fabric panel which has a large surface area, and is therefore not excessively restrictive to airflow. They are compatible with most furnaces and central air conditioners, though adaptations to the sheet metal work may be needed. It is best to use the largest size which can be made to fit in the available space.

Bag-type and box-type extended media filters have medium to high efficiency and medium to high resistance to air flow. These are commonly used in special air-cleaning systems, portable filters and with fan-coil forced-air systems equipped with high-pressure fans. See the Heating section in 79 Best Healthy Building Solutions. A wide range of efficiencies is available in these types, up to hospital clean-room standard. The most efficient are capable of trapping pollens, fungal spores, fine soil and some bacteria in the one micron range (one-thousandth of a millimeter).

HEPA, extended media (high efficiency particulate arrestance) is an advanced type of fabric filter. These have very high efficiency and very high resistance to air flow. They are commonly used in hospital and industrial clean-room situations, and in high-performance portable air cleaners or custom filter systems. The biological grade is capable of trapping bacteria as well as other very fine particles. They are up to 99.9% efficient for 0.3 micron particles.

Electronic and Electrostatic Filters

Electronic filters have high efficiency and moderate resistance to airflow. They do not contain porous fabric, but have metal grids which are charged by a high-voltage electrical supply. The charge causes particles to be attracted to the grid where they can be removed by periodic cleaning. These units are very effective in forced-air systems, but require regular care. They may become noisy, ineffective or produce small amounts of irritating ozone if not serviced properly. The manufacturer's instructions for servicing should be followed closely. Passive electrostatic filters are another type of filter alternative. They use no electricity, but contain a grid of plastic wires which become statically charged by the airflow over them. They are not as effective as electronic filters or medium-efficiency, pleated and bag filters, but are better than standard furnace filters.

Filter Ratings

There are three filter efficiency rating methods as defined by ASHRAE (American Society of Heating, Refrigeration, and Air Conditioning Engineers). These are the Arrestance Method, the Atmospheric Dust Spot, and the D.O.P. Method.

The Arrestance Method is not very useful and should not be referred to for the primary air filters in a healthy building. Filter manufacturers who use this method for furnace filters are providing misleading efficiency ratings and should be avoided. This method is only useful for very coarse filters, such as those in a kitchen exhaust.

The Atmospheric Dust Spot Method is the usual reference test for household forced-air filters. Over 20% efficiency by this method is "medium efficiency." Anything over 40% is a good target for the primary filter in a healthy building.

The D.O.P. Method is only used for very high-performance filters, such as HEPA filters used in special air cleaners. See the Air Filter Efficiency table in 79 Best Healthy Building Solutions for more details.

Odor Filters

Odor and volatile gas removal is performed by a special type of filter called an adsorption filter. An adsorption material is one which contains microscopic pores able to trap gases and hold them until they can be disposed of. Activated carbon and crystalline zeolite are common types of adsorbent material.

Activated Carbon (charcoal)

Activated carbon is the most common and broadly effective gas adsorption material. It is effective for many solvent odors, diesel and other fuel odors, alcohol odors, body and bathroom odors, cooking odors, dry cleaning odors, paint and adhesive odors and pet odors. It is not highly effective for formaldehyde, ammonia and some irritating components of urban smog, such as sulfur and nitrogen oxides. Activated carbon is usually made from wood, coconut shell, coal or peat, by treating it at very high temperatures.

Carbon in the form of pellets or flakes is used in a thin filter frame made with a metal screen. The frames may be refillable, and usually require a change two to four times per year. These have a high resistance to airflow, however, and can only be used with a high-pressure fan, such as the type used in a good-quality portable air cleaner. It is possible to add a carbon pellet filter to a forced-air heating or air conditioning system, but it is usually done in a "bypass" configuration, either with or without a separate fan. The reason for this is that the resistance to air flow is too great to accept the entire flow of most systems. See the Ventilating section in 79 Best Healthy Building Solutions.

Carbon-treated fabric is also available as a pleated, medium-efficiency

A standard furnace filter is not adequate for the healthy home.

filter. The carbon in these filters has been powdered and mixed into the fabric. These can accept the full airflow from a forced-air system, but are not as effective at trapping gases as the pellet carbon is, and will need to be changed more often in polluted circumstances because the amount of carbon is very small.

Zeolite

Zeolite is a mineral mined from porous stone deposits. Like carbon, it contains microscopic pores which trap gases. It is particularly effective for ammonia odors from pets and urine spills. Zeolite is not a substitute for carbon for general odor removal purposes, but can be an important supplement.

Warning: Adsorption filters will usually collect moisture quite readily, and begin to deteriorate if used in damp locations. They should only be used in a dry air stream which is relatively free of particles and oily substances. This usually requires protecting them with a fabric prefilter.

Reactive Scrubbers

Reactive scrubbers react chemically with gases and render them inert or stable until they can be disposed of. Potassium permanganate on a base of activated alumina is a common type of reactive scrubber material. It is particularly effective for formaldehyde and hydrogen sulfide (rotten egg odor).

Other specialized scrubbers can be used in situations where specific irritants are identified which cannot be avoided, such as in a photo lab, printing shop or other situation. A custom filter can be prepared for identified air contaminants, using two or more filter media together. This work must be done by a qualified filtration consultant.

Filter Location and Fan Operation

Air filters are most effective when they receive a recirculated air stream, such as the filter in a forced-air furnace, or a central or portable room air cleaner. Trapping particles or gases in a filter is a matter of chance, so the more times contaminated air is passed through a filter, the better the chance of trapping contaminants. However, filters are sometimes used in single-pass locations, such as outdoor air supply ducts. In this case the efficiency of the filter becomes critical, since there will only be one chance to trap contaminants.

All forced-air filters also work better with a continuous fan operation, now common in newer heating and air conditioning equipment. The fan runs constantly on low speed to maintain air filtration. It switches to high speed only when heating or cooling is needed.

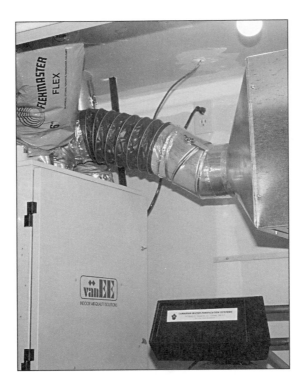

A particle and odor removal filter bank installed in a ventilator intake in an urban location where air quality is poor.

Activated carbon is the most broadly effective odor removal filter.

Filter Restriction to Air Flow

All filters present some resistance to the flow of air, and as they become loaded the resistance increases. It is critically important that filter resistance be matched to the equipment in which it is used. If resistance is too high for the fan, the filter and the equipment will not perform effectively. This is particularly important for high-efficiency filters and for filter upgrades for forced-air heating and ventilation systems. This should be determined by a qualified heating and ventilation contractor or consultant. Often a high-resistance type of filter can be added to a forced-air or ventilating system, but it will have to be large enough to minimize reaction. This may require extra sheet metal work in the system.

One reason that electronic filters are so popular for air cleaners and furnace upgrades is that they present relatively little resistance to air flow, yet provide medium- to high-efficiency performance.

Filter Materials

The environmentally hypersensitive must be cautious about the type of material they choose for a filter. Some fabrics and fibers may have a slight odor or release small amounts of irritating dust. The most common materials for low- and medium-efficiency filters are polyester or spun-glass mats or fabrics. These are generally made with small amounts of adhesive or binders to hold them together and they may be coated with oily or sticky materials to make them more effective. Polyester fabrics themselves are generally not odorous, nor are glass fibers, but glass fibers may release irritating particles when handled. For those few affected by these materials, polyester-cotton blends or all-cotton fabric filters are available in medium-efficiency types, and may be more acceptable. Some high-efficiency filters are made from filter paper, or cellulose-glass paper blends, which are usually acceptable to the hypersensitive. They are generally made from very pure materials with no coatings. These are often used in very high-performance air cleaners with box-type filters. The types listed as "wet laid" usually contain less binder. Air freshener additives can be avoided by selecting the filters which do not use them, but there is some adhesive used in nearly all filter construction. For extremely sensitive persons, custom filters made with sewn (stitched) fabric may be necessary.

Hypersensitive persons may also find that the source of the carbons used in a carbon filter makes a difference to them. Several types should be tested by sniffing, and running brief trials in the air filter system to determine which type is tolerated best.

WATER

Water Quality in the Healthy Home

Water quality is an essential element in the healthy home. Many people today are justifiably concerned about the quality of both rural and municipal water supplies. Raw water supplied to municipal plants from surface sources has been declining in quality for many years, particularly in densely populated and heavily industrialized areas. Consequently, chemical treatment is also accelerating. Many who rely on local ground water are also faced with contamination by agricultural and industrial waste, and are buying bottled drinking water or installing home water treatment systems because they do not trust their water supply. Many people who have chlorinated tap water from a municipal system, use bottled water for drinking and cooking, not necessarily due to health concerns but simply because it tastes so much better.

The actual health risk from drinking water is probably highest for those who are served by local or rural water supplies from wells or surface water. This water is the most likely to be contaminated by sewage, animal droppings, agricultural chemicals or industrial chemicals. However, not all water quality problems are created by human activity. Excessive hardness (mineral content), metal content, salt content and hydrogen sulfide are some of the common, naturally occurring problems which have always existed. Due to the possibility of contamination from all sources, water from a local supply *not* regulated by a water district should be tested before it is used. Some treatment, including sterilization to remove parasites and hazardous bacteria, is often necessary. Thereafter the water should be tested as often as annually, depending on the risk of contamination of the source. Your local health department can provide advice on testing.

Water supplied by a municipal district is likely to be relatively free of bacteria, parasites and industrial chemicals (though accidental contamination does sometimes occur), but it has a different set of problems caused by the treatment and piping systems. The filtration plant may use chemicals which leave aluminum and other residues in water, and the system is almost certain to be treated with chlorine to control bacteria and parasites. All municipal, raw water supplies from surface sources contain some organic materials, usually from rotting vegetation, soil erosion in watersheds and leaky pipes. When chlorine is added to control bacteria, it combines with the organic materials and produces irritating and potentially hazardous substances, such as methyl chloroform. The volatile substances from chlorination are obviously ingested through drinking, but are absorbed equally by showering, because they are atomized in the showerhead and then inhaled. Chlorine also tends to corrode metal pipes and fittings, adding more contaminants to the water.

Not all filter fabrics will be acceptable to those with sensitivities.

Determining Water Treatment Needs

The first task in successful water treatment is to determine what, if any, treatment is necessary. Water contaminants must be identified, and the treatment must be specifically designed for the conditions. Fortunately, unlike air quality problems, which can be very difficult to identify by testing, water quality testing is a relatively simple and inexpensive procedure. A basic water test for coliform bacteria, minerals, metals and salt is routine and costs about $25 to $50. If you are on a municipal system, these tests are required periodically, and the results can be obtained from your local water authority. If other local contaminants are suspected, such as agricultural chemicals or industrial waste, more sophisticated tests can be done which can identify several hundred other contaminants. These tests are expensive, however, and should be ordered by a qualified public health professional or water quality consultant. In some cases, a regional health authority or environmental agency will do the testing, particularly if several households are affected.

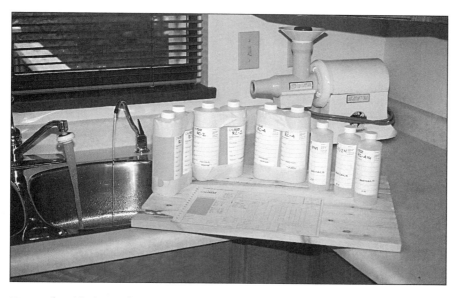

Water should always be tested or a water quality report obtained from your water district before deciding on treatment.

Water Purification Systems and Equipment

There are two basic types of water purification systems: point-of-use systems and whole house systems. The point-of-use system is one which treats the water only at one location in the home. The system may treat it as it passes through the tap or shower, or it may deliver it to a small storage container and then to a special tap, which is usually installed in the kitchen. This tap is then used for drinking and cooking. A whole house system treats water before it enters the home plumbing, and may treat all the water, or just that which flows to the kitchen and bathrooms. There is usually no treatment done for water used in the yard and garden.

Countertop, point-of-use systems can be installed by connection to a tap, requiring no plumbing changes. Built-in point-of-use or whole house water treatment systems can usually be added to existing plumbing if the pipes are accessible, but a plumber will be needed. In the healthy home, when installing new plumbing, or for new construction, it is a good idea to allow space and plumbing connections for water treatment systems, even if they will not be installed immediately. Some systems also require an electrical supply and a drain for the discharge of water diverted past the filters, or used for occasional backwashing. This should be considered when planning an installation.

There are several basic types of water treatment. Each is able to remove only some contaminants.

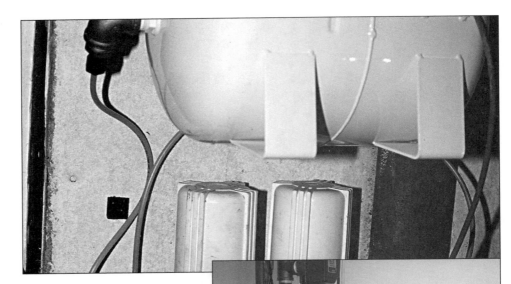

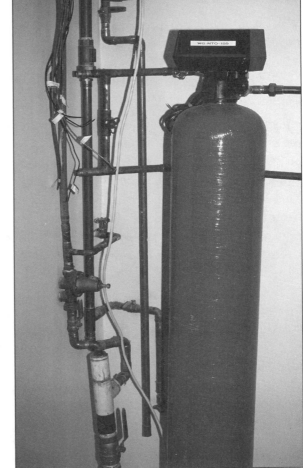

A whole house carbon treatment system.

A point-of-use reuse osmosis and carbon treatment system.

You must know what you are treating for before deciding on water treatment methods.

166

Sediment removal

These are basically fine sieve filters, usually in the form of disposable cartridges made from polyester or mineral-fiber fabric tightly woven around a plastic core. When water is forced through these under pressure, small particles are trapped in the fabric. Common sediment filters are effective for particles of about five microns (five-thousandths of a millimeter) and larger. This makes them capable of trapping most soil, sand, rust and coarse organic materials. These do not generally produce excessive restriction to water flow, and, if large enough, can be used in whole house filters. A sediment filter should always be used where water is often cloudy, and also to protect more delicate filtration equipment, such as reverse osmosis or carbon units, from sediment blockage. Sediments are primarily an esthetic and housekeeping problem, they are usually not a health risk, unless they contain untreated runoff which may carry bacteria or parasites. Fine filters, capable of trapping one micron particles, are also available, but are much larger and more expensive than five micron filters, especially for whole house use.

Mineral removal

Hard water is a common problem in many areas, particularly where ground water is drawn from limestone formations. Hardness is caused by dissolved calcium carbonate mineral, though other minerals may be involved. Hardness is generally only a nuisance because it stains fixtures, makes soap ineffective and plugs pipes. Water softening is done by softener systems using a tank containing an ion-exchange resin, which attracts minerals. The tank is then periodically flushed with salt, which removes the trapped minerals and restores the resin. Though high mineral content is not usually considered a health risk, the unavoidable salt residue introduced by the softener after replenishing may be a risk to those on low-sodium diets. Softened water should not be used regularly for drinking or cooking, only for bathing and laundry.

Sterilization

Surface water or ground water contaminated by sewage or animal waste has a high risk of carrying fecal coliform bacteria and other disease-causing organisms, such as amoebas, cryptosporidium and giardia. This risk is considered the major public health problem with water systems. Municipal water should be relatively free of these problems, but rural systems may require in-home sterilization.

The usual method is a small ultraviolet lamp which contacts the water

167

stream before use. Ultraviolet light effectively destroys harmful organisms if it is strong enough, and the contact time is long enough. Unlike chlorination, this process leaves no hazardous residue in the water. It is also possible to use ozone injection in a similar way. Ultraviolet sterilizers are not effective in all situations, however. For example, sediments in water will coat the lamp and reduce its effectiveness. Particles may also carry attached bacteria and parasites past the lamp without exposing them to ultraviolet. For this reason, a good sediment filter is necessary before water enters the sterilization chambers. A qualified water quality consultant should design the system if sterilization is necessary.

Metal removal

Water supplies occasionally contain quantities of metals, such as iron or magnesium, which are mainly nuisances, or sometimes more toxic metals, such as lead, mercury or cadmium. Treatment systems similar to water softeners (above), using an ion exchange resin, may be used for removal of some metals, or specialized chemical methods may be used. Some metal removal is also accomplished by reverse osmosis (see salt removal and organic compound removal below). Generally, where serious metal problems exist, a treatment system may be required designed specifically for local conditions. A water quality consultant should be used in these circumstances.

Dechlorinating

Removing chlorine and chlorine products from municipal water is a common procedure in healthy housing. These contaminants affect the taste of the water, and are irritants to those with sensitivities. Most health authorities also acknowledge that they are actually a small health risk for any population.

The most common method of removal is with an "activated carbon" pellet or carbon block system. Carbon contains microscopic pores which are able to trap many contaminants in water, improving its taste and odor. Carbon treatment is effective, whether used as a whole house system or at point-of-use. The most important factors for an effective carbon system are the quantity of carbon contained in it, and the amount of contact time the water has with it. Only systems with large volumes of carbon are effective for large flows. A shower filter or kitchen tap filter can be effective with about one pound of carbon (450 grams), but a full-flow, whole house system should have much more, usually over five pounds (2.2 kilograms). Once chlorine has been removed, however, water is again prone to microbial contamination. If it must stand in the pipes for lengthy periods, an ultraviolet sterilization unit should be added (see sterilization above).

Water supplied from wells or local surface sources is much more likely to present health problems.

Salt removal

Reverse osmosis systems are the most popular for salt removal. These units force water, under pressure, through a polyester membrane. Most contaminants are left behind because they will not pass through the membrane. The process is slow, however, so a large storage tank is required for the fresh water supply to the kitchen or house. The process also wastes a good deal of water, because it requires a continuous flow past the membrane to prevent it from clogging. About four to six units of bypass water are discharged to a drain for every unit treated.

Reverse osmosis elements are most common in under-sink systems, though countertop units are also available. Whole house reverse osmosis units are available, but are very complex and expensive. A small, countertop distillation unit can also be used to remove salt, but these use a lot of electricity, and produce small amounts of water.

Organic compound removal

Reverse osmosis units, described above for salt removal, are also used for organic compound removal and can serve a kitchen or whole house. Organic compounds are either odorous substances from soil or vegetation, or chemicals from industry or agriculture. Carbon filtering, described above for removal of chlorine compounds, is also used for organic compound removal, but should be preceded by a reverse osmosis filter if contamination is serious. Otherwise the carbon will not be fully effective and will become contaminated too quickly.

Buffering

In some situations the water is acidic due to its source. This may occur in watersheds with acidic soil, or where acid rain is severe. Acidic water is always very soft, and will leach metals such as lead and copper from plumbing, stain fixtures and reduce the life of the pipes. A whole house buffering unit can be used to reduce acidity of the water to alleviate these problems. It consists of a tank containing an alkaline material, usually ground limestone, which converts some of the acidity of the water on contact. These add a small amount of hardness (calcium carbonate) to the water, but not enough to require softening. The buffer material must be renewed periodically as it is consumed. The buffer can be added to a carbon whole house treatment system, where needed.

Equipment Cost

The least costly water treatment units are point-of-use carbon filters, such as countertop units, under-counter units, or shower filters for chlorine removal. These are available for $50 to $200 US. The most important considerations are the amount of carbon contained in the unit, and the cost of carbon replacement. As a consumer, be cautious about very inexpensive units that are either not refillable, or have expensive, "special" replacement cartridges. Special cartridges will end up costing much more than a bulk refillable unit which can be refilled by the user, or standard cartridges. Countertop distillation units which can treat and sterilize small quantities of kitchen water cost about $150 to $300 US.

A more sophisticated point-of-use unit, either for under counter or countertop use, containing a prefilter, a reverse osmosis filter and a small storage tank, followed by a carbon filter, costs about $300 to $800 US, depending on size and features.

The cost of whole house filters varies widely, depending on the treatment requirements and the capacity of the filter. A whole house carbon unit for chlorine removal, made from basic water softener hardware (without the softener resin replaced by carbon and a sand filter) will cost about $1000 US including installation. It may also contain a buffer, if the water is acidic. Replacing the buffer and carbon costs about $50 to $100 US. Other whole house systems for softening and simple metal removal are in the same price range. A whole house salt removal system, or other specialized system using a large reverse osmosis membrane or chemical contact tanks and storage tanks, may cost several thousand dollars, including pumps, tanks and wiring.

Equipment Maintenance

All water treatment equipment requires periodic maintenance and replacement of disposable filters and bulk media. This is particularly important with units using carbon filters because these will become contaminated over time and may support hazardous bacteria. Replacement of smaller sediment filters and carbon units in point-of-use systems is usually necessary at least twice a year. Larger units, such as whole house carbon filters, may only require replacement carbon every two years. Reverse osmosis elements will need occasional replacement (from 3 to 10 years), depending on what quantities of contaminants reach them. It is very important to have a good sediment filter in front of a reverse osmosis or carbon filter in order to protect it, and to change the sediment filter regularly to maintain the required flow.

If you install any sophisticated water treatment equipment, it is usually best to trust servicing to a qualified service contractor. Often service can be purchased for a reasonable annual fee.

Reverse osmosis units are effective for salt and organic compound removal, but they waste a good deal of water.

CHAPTER 9

Materials

MATERIALS SELECTION

Healthy materials are those which have a minimum of offgassing potential, minimum potential to trap or release dust, and a minimum ability to trap odors. They must also be individually acceptable.

Healthy material choices can be successfully made by a combination of research, rules of avoidance and experience. There are presently very few useful standards for healthy materials, but there is a growing body of research which can help. If the healthy design is intended for a very sensitive individual, however, much more rigor and caution must be used for materials selection. For these cases, it is best to get expert advice from a consultant with specialized experience.

The advice on healthy materials in this book is "generic," that is, it is based on classes or categories of materials, not on specific products by trade name. The generic approach offered here can help to set priorities, and to make basic decisions. More detailed decisions will usually depend on the specific project.

Though there can be important variations between different manufacturers in some industries, the generic approach is useful for products such as manufactured woods, paints, cabinet construction materials and hard floor coverings. It is not as useful in other categories, such as carpets, where differences between manufacturers and even between different production runs by the same manufacturer may be great.

Another consideration is setting priorities, because not all materials are equally important for health. To determine which materials are the highest priority for selection, key points to consider are:

- *Quantity:* How much of the material will be exposed to indoor air? (Floor and wall coverings cover large indoor areas, for instance.)
- *Location:* How close will the material be to occupants or the air

handling system? (Furniture and bedding are close to occupants, and duct materials are in contact with ventilation air.)

- *Duration:* How long are emissions expected to continue? (Finishes with highly volatile contents such as lacquer have short-term emissions; others with semi-volatile contents such as oil paints and carpets have long-term emissions.)
- *Emissions:* What gases and dusts are likely to be emitted into the air from the product during installation and in use, and to what extent will it adsorb and release odors and trap soil? (Some materials, such as soft plastics, are "known emitters," while others, such as ceramics, are very inert and unlikely to adsorb gases or trap soils.)
- *Toxicity:* What hazard level is presented by the gases and dusts emitted? (Some are irritants, some neurotoxins and some are potential carcinogens. Those with the highest risk are listed on Material Safety Data Sheets.)
- *Occupancy:* Will the building be occupied when the emissions are occurring? (It is relatively easy to provide approved respirators for protection of tradespeople, but difficult to completely isolate work areas in occupied buildings.)
- *Durability:* How much is the material likely to break down during its service life? (Textiles and many soft plastics deteriorate with time, especially when exposed to ultraviolet light, while metals, glass, ceramics and many woods do not.)
- *Maintenance requirements:* How much cleaning, waxing, stain resistance treatment, refinishing and other high-impact maintenance will it require in place? (Many cleaning and sealing procedures for interior finishes introduce volatile materials, including some toxic solvents.)

These considerations will lead to a "most significant contributors" list for the project. This list should set priorities for low-emission materials selection. Often, floor, wall and ceiling coverings, cabinets and furniture materials, and filter and duct materials are the highest priorities.

Materials are a particular concern at three distinct times in their life cycle:

- *Installation:* What will be the exposure of tradespeople and building occupants during construction or renovation? This information can be found in Material Safety Data Sheets (see below).
- *Occupant exposure:* What will be the exposure of building occupants to materials emissions during building use?
- *Maintenance and removal:* What will be the exposure of building

occupants and tradespeople during maintenance procedures and removal or demolition?

In making health-based decisions, it has been common to accept short-term health risks during installation in exchange for long-term benefits. For example, solvent-based finishes such as lacquers are risky to handle, but often very safe and durable when cured. Fortunately, due to increasing environmental regulation and changing industrial processes, it is now possible to find many materials which protect both the health of the installer and the building user, and are produced with reduced environmental impact. New acrylic-latex interior paints and low volatile-content adhesives are good examples of products combining good performance and durability with low toxicity to the user and the environment.

But there are still tradeoffs to be made. For example, sanding and finishing a wood floor is very messy, and somewhat toxic. But after cleanup and curing of the finish, it is a very healthy floor.

Generic Materials Selection

New materials indoors are sources of volatile gases and dusts, which are important air pollutants. Aging materials, such as soiled carpets and upholstery, are also sources of dust and odors. A few simple rules will help to guide selection practice toward healthier choices.

- Minimize the use of standard particle boards and interior plywoods. These formaldehyde sources are common as flooring underlay and in inexpensive cabinets and furniture. Use exterior grade plywoods and, if particle board is necessary, look for low-emission products, such as those bearing the European E1 or the U.S. HUD label. Completely formaldehyde-free MDF (medium density fiberboard), is available from specialty wood suppliers.
- Select acrylic and latex paints and adhesives meeting the New Jersey or California air quality standards and bearing the "zero VOC" label.
- Use prefinished materials wherever possible to minimize sanding and finishing in place. For example, factory-finished wood flooring and millwork are widely available.
- Minimize the use of soft plastics, such as sheet vinyl floor coverings. These have prolonged emissions.
- Minimize the use of fixed carpets. Hard floors, such as wood and ceramics, with area rugs are best for low emissions and easy maintenance.
- Minimize the use of exposed acoustic surfaces and fabric coverings, drapery, non-washable upholstery, etc.

173

PERSONAL CHALLENGE TESTING

Your own senses are exquisite instruments which are meant to alert you to your environment. With careful attention, you can learn to judge healthy materials, or find problems such as mildew, dust, or volatile emissions in items such as paints, cleaners, glues and carpets. In some ways, your nose, eyes, skin and immune system can tell you more than a sophisticated laboratory instrument can. Before selecting a home, a school or an office, pay attention to how it affects you. How does it smell, when you first arrive? First impressions can tell a lot. How do the surfaces look? Are they dusty? Does it seem well maintained?

Check around thoroughly, looking in enclosed areas, under furniture and cabinets, in the basement, and in any moist areas. Check any crawl space or the attic space if possible. Remember that your nose becomes fatigued quickly. If you go outside again every few minutes, you can refresh your ability to smell, then go back in. However, if outdoor air is very polluted, this won't be effective.

When choosing materials, your observations are very useful, particularly if you are highly sensitive. Samples of the material can be brought into close contact with your nose and face, and touched against the skin of the forearm, at first just briefly. If this proves acceptable, try them for a few minutes to determine if there is any adverse reaction. The sample will have to be large enough and fresh enough to reasonably simulate actual conditions of exposure. For example, a fabric or wood sample should be at least one square foot. Liquid finishes such as paint may be applied to a nonemitting surface, such as metal or glass, and allowed to cure for a few days, then checked closely for odors and reactions.

Many materials which cause adverse reactions will have a detectable odor, but some do not, or their odor is too subtle to detect immediately or from a small sample. Another useful test, particularly for fabrics, paints, wood products and floor coverings, is to place a small sample in a clean glass jar with a metal lid. Seal it tightly, and keep it in a warm area, or in the sun for a day. Any emissions from the material will collect in the jar and be more detectable when the jar is opened. Those with sensitive skin will also wish to pretest fabrics by placing a small strip against the skin, in an area such as the inside of the forearm. Wrap the strip all the way around, and use a safety pin to hold it together. Be sure the fabric is fully washed, rinsed and dried. Some people with sensitivities find that several washings in a baking soda or borax solution, followed by several rinses, helps to remove factory sizing and other contaminants from fabric. An hour of contact with the skin should reveal any sensitivity problems. This test is particularly important for clothing, bedding and upholstery materials.

Once you have determined which materials are the most likely choices, try living with them for a while, one at a time. Keep a large sample by your bed, or in the case of fabrics, under your pillow for a few days.

This book offers materials selection advice for healthy buildings and interiors and this advice is reliable for most people, but safe materials are ultimately an individual matter, particularly for the environmentally sensitive person. For the sensitive person, the safety of each material must be carefully assessed before it is used. An experienced physician or environmental consultant can assist with testing.

MATERIAL SAFETY DATA SHEETS

Every manufacturer of a product which may have health and safety implications in the workplace is required by law to provide a Material Safety Data Sheet (MSDS) on request. The sheet provides a summary of the chemical composition of a material (though manufacturers are not required to list certain ingredients which are protected trade secrets), including health risks, flammability, and handling and storage precautions. Manufacturers must disclose the presence of any contents which are listed as carcinogens, potent caustics, explosives, or are high risk for other reasons. Though an MSDS is a technical document, requiring some chemistry and health knowledge to read accurately, a great deal can be learned from it by anyone. MSDS information on paints, varnishes, waxes, glues and cleaners, for example, can provide a basis for comparison, even for the lay reader. Where a more technical analysis is required, you may know someone with workplace safety training who can assist with interpretation of the data sheets.

Some of the key concepts used in MSDS are:

Carcinogenic Classifications

These state whether the contents of the product are listed as potential or likely causes of cancer. The usual categories are None (no risk known), Listed (risk potential), Potential (established potential), Probable (high-risk potential), or Known (well-established risk).

TLV (Threshold Limit Value)

This is the accepted toxicity threshold for breathing a hazardous material. The lower the TLV, the more toxic the agent is.

Typical units: ppm (parts per million) or mg/m^3 (milligrams per cubic meter of air).

TWA (Time Weighted Average)

This is the allowable exposure limit for breathing material over a working day, usually eight hours. The lower the TWA, the more toxic the agent is.

Typical units: ppm or mg/m^3.

PEL (Permissible Exposure Limit)

This is the maximum exposure allowed for industrial handling. An "R" indicates respiratory and an "S" indicates skin absorption.

Typical units: ppm or mg/m^3.

TVOC (Total Volatile Organic Content)

This states the volume of the product which will evaporate over time. The higher the TVOC the more the product adds to indoor pollution. This rating indicates products which may be labeled "low VOC" or "zero VOC."

Typical units: % or gms/liter

Some other useful concepts for interpreting Material Safety Data Sheets:

Vapor Pressure

This is the pressure produced by evaporation of the volatile contents of a material. The higher the vapor pressure the more rapidly the volatile contents will evaporate.

Typical units: mm.Hg (millimeters of mercury).

Mineral Fiber Content

This states the presence of potentially respirable mineral fibers which can be released during handling or use. This is especially important for insulations and acoustic tiles.

NFPA Heath Risk Number

The NFPA (National Fire Protection Association) has developed a system of classification of risk, primarily for the protection of firefighters. The NFPA method gives three numbers, for Flammability, Reactivity, and Health. The numbers range from 0 to 4. A product health-rated as a 0 can be assumed to be very low in hazardous emissions, while a product rated as a 4 is obviously dangerous to handle. This rating can tell you quite a lot.

When renovating an occupied building, the safety of interior products is paramount. The safest paints, adhesives, other coatings and caulkings are rated a 0 or a 1 on the NFPA or equivalent health-rating scale. However, a few products with a high health risk are highly volatile and are safe once cured. Sanding sealer for wood finishing is a good example.

Many mineral ingredients in paints or panel products, such as mineral fiber or silica, are listed as hazardous, though they may be highly contained within the material and unlikely to be released. This type of warning does indicate that spraying panels or sanding or cutting with power tools should be avoided, because it would release the mineral contents.

Common Abbreviations

ACGIH—American Conference of Governmental Industrial Hygienists
CCOHS—Canadian Centre for Occupational Health and Safety
CAS—Chemical Abstracts Services
N.D.—None Detected
IARC—International Agency for Research on Cancer
NIOSH—National Institute of Occupational Safety and Health
NOEL—No Observable Effect Level
NTP—National Toxicology Program
OHSA—Occupational Health and Safety Administration
SARA—Superfund Amendments Reauthorization Act
TSCA—Toxic Substances Control Act
VOC—Volatile Organic Compound
WHMIS—Workplace Hazardous Materials Information System

LD50 (Lethal Dose, 50%)

This is the dose which is lethal to 50% of laboratory animals when ingested. The lower the LD50, the more toxic the agent is when ingested.

Typical units: mg/kg (body weight).

LC50 (Lethal Concentration, 50%)

This is the concentration of the agent in air which is lethal to 50% of laboratory animals when breathed. The lower the LC50, the more toxic the agent is when inhaled.

Typical units: ppm or mg/m^3.

Polymerization

This is the ability of a substance to react rapidly with air or other substances causing heat, flame or explosion.

CHECKLIST OF HEALTHY MATERIALS AND SYSTEMS

AVOID	PREFERRED

Site

Industrial areas; mechanized agriculture (sprays and fertilizers); highways; low-lying ground (dampness, stagnant air, insects and flood risk); extreme weather exposure; poor sunlight and daylight exposure; allergenic grasses, shrubs and trees; large power lines, substations and local power distribution equipment.

Residential areas; semi-rural areas; "high and dry" sites; access to fresh breezes and light; shelter from extreme sun and storms; deciduous trees and less allergenic plants near site (based on individual sensitivities).

Soils and Soil Treatment

Landfill sites; heavy clay; standing water; powdery dust; residual pesticide treatment for termites, ants, etc.

Well-drained, sandy loam; vegetation ground cover; physical pest control barriers.

Excavation and Drainage

Buried topsoil; clay spread on surface; inadequate drainage of excavation to lower ground; soil sloped toward building, low-quality drainage pipes, asphalt foundation damp-proofing; imported topsoil with unknown history.

Topsoil separated for reuse; clay removed from site; soil sloped away from foundations; high-capacity, durable drainage system (designed for local climate); cementitious type, damp-proofing, drainage membranes, porous foundation insulation, clean gravel backfill.

Concrete and Forms

Inadequate steel reinforcing, super-plasticizer concrete additives; concrete water-reducing agents; other oil-based concrete additives; diesel or motor oil form release.

Engineered reinforcing plain cement/sand/gravel mixes, vegetable oil or unscented mineral oil form release.

Masonry

Masonry, stone, block and brick foundations in wet conditions; masonry foundations below four feet deep; brick facing without adequate air space and drainage courses; masonry walls without adequate insulation (cold climates).

Above-ground masonry; insulated wall sheathing behind masonry; plain cement/lime/sand mortar for indoor masonry; silicone, acrylic, or waterglass (sodium silicate) sealer to reduce dust and moisture absorption (where required).

Carpentry

Pressure-treated woods (especially where people walk or sit); engineered wood products with interior glues (UF Glue); engineered wood products with high glue contents (e.g. strand board, particle board); anti-sapstain treated softwoods; large amounts of allergenic softwoods indoors (based on individual sensitivity).

Rot-resistant construction details; rot-resistant woods; plastic lumber sill plates and deck components; solid woods; exterior plywoods (PF Glue); formaldehyde-free particle board (where individually acceptable); hardwood or sealed softwood interior details, with low-toxicity finishes.

Thermal and Moisture Protection

Roofing

Tar and gravel roofs; rubber membrane roofs; wood shingle roofs in very wet climates, or less than 20-degree slope; asbestos shingles; low-quality, asphalt shingles.

Torch-on (oxidized) asphalt membrane (where flat roofs are necessary); cement tile or wood fiber/cement shingles; galvanized steel; fiberglass reinforced asphalt shingles.

Cladding

Stucco systems in wet weather exposures; asbestos siding; wood less than 12 inches (30 cm) off ground (prone to termites and rot); wood requiring regular painting.

Stone or brick; tile; wood fiber/cement panels or shingles; stucco or adobe in dry locations; plated metals; natural wood (with weather-protective finish, as needed).

AVOID	PREFERRED

Weather barrier (on outside of walls)

Fresh, asphalt-treated paper; untreated paper; no weather barrier in exposed locations; impermeable plastic or closed-cell plastic foam insulation.	Polyolefin weather barrier; perforated plastic weather barrier, air-permeable insulation board.

Insulation

Urea formaldehyde foam (UFFI); loose fill mineral products (vermiculite, perlite); plastic foams exposed to indoors; any leaky insulation cavities.	Cotton insulation; loose fill cellulose fiber; wood fiber boards; fiber-safe glass or mineral fiber batts without adhesive binder or with latex adhesive (specialty products).

Air vapor barrier (on warm side of insulation)

No air vapor barrier with highly insulated wall and ceiling; air leakage paths into insulated spaces; perforated air vapor barrier; solvent caulkings used for installation.	Airtight drywall or plaster system; foil barrier, taped seams; polyethylene barrier, taped seams.

Windows and Light
Daylight

Large evergreen trees or adjacent buildings obstructing sky in cloudy climates; tinted glass in cloudy climates; excessive, unsheltered glass in clear sky climates.	Open view of sky in cloudy climates; sheltered view of sky in clear sky climates; good balance of north, east and south exposures; sheltered west exposure; clear glass; north and east windows and skylights.

Solar control

Limited access to winter sun in cold climates; limited shelter from sun in warm climates; west exposure only; large skylights facing south or west.	Leafy trees on south and west; shading overhangs for summer shelter; limited windows to west; attached sunspace for winter.

Cross-ventilation

Very limited opening windows; all opening windows on one side; all opening windows low on the wall; opening windows close to busy streets, damp or pollen-bearing vegatation near windows.

Opening windows on two or three sides of major rooms (6% of floor area); low inlet windows and high outlet windows.

Doors

Particle board core doors; vinyl-coated or woodgrain interior plywood doors; old doors with lead paint.

Solid wood doors; glass doors; solid wood with glass doors; enameled metal doors.

Interior Finishes
Walls

Vinyl-coated or woodgrain interior plywood; heavily flocked wallpaper; rough or unfinished wood paneling; badly deteriorating plaster; chronically moisture-damaged surfaces.

Traditional plaster (lime/gypsum/sand); cement plaster (white cement, sand and lime); gypsum wallboard, painted both sides (see Paints); concrete or masonry; smooth wallpaper; exterior plywood or fiber cement board; fully finished, solid woods; porcelain panels.

Ceilings

Badly deteriorating plaster; heavily perforated acoustic tile; rough or unfinished wood.

Traditional plaster (lime/gypsum/sand); cement plaster (white cement, sand, lime); patterned metal panels; gypsum wallboard, painted both sides (see Paints); fully finished, solid woods.

Paints and varnishes

Old, lead-based paint; using oil-based paints, solvent lacquers and varnishes in occupied buildings; acid-curing oil finishes containing formaldehyde; latex paints in

Low-emission (zero VOCs) acrylic latex paints; linseed oil, hardening type oil finishes; water-dispersed urethanes and acrylics; other low-toxicity, clear sealers; beeswax or

181

AVOID	PREFERRED
chronically damp locations; exterior or industrial paints indoors; heavily tinted paints, except zero VOCs or "all natural" formulations.	carnauba wax finishes; factory-cured finishes, e.g. urethanes, powder coatings and enamels.

Floors

New, soft vinyl flooring; new, latex-bonded carpet; (except special low-emissions constructions) deep pile carpet; soiled carpet or carpet in damp areas; rubber-type carpet cushion; refinishing wood floors in occupied buildings; plastic or asphalt-type flooring adhesives; petroleum solvent, based tile and stone sealers;	Ceramic or stone floors, set in cement mortar; finished concrete floors; factory-finished hardwoods, nailed or floating; linseed oil linoleum, sealed; reinforced vinyl tile, sealed; washable throw rugs.

Bath enclosures

New fiberglass or acrylic molded units; plastic doors; many joints requiring caulking; plastic tile adhesives; fiber cement backer boards with chemical curing agents; waterproof gypsum board tile backers.	Enamel steel, china or cast iron fixtures; glass and metal doors; ceramic tile set in cement mortar; glass tile set in silicone; sealed tile grouts with water-resistant low-toxicity sealers.

Furnishings
Upholstery fabric

New vinyl or leather covers; stain- and crease-resistant treatments; rough fabrics in contact with skin (depending on sensitivities); very porous covers.	Untreated cottons; washable cotton/ synthetic blends; wool (if tolerated), dust barrier cloth covers (300 threads per inch).

Upholstery fillings

Feathers (down), kapok and hair (depending on allergies); new chipped foam or rubber; perfumed treatments.	Cotton batting; polyester fiber or wool (depending on allergies); metal springs.

AVOID	PREFERRED

Cabinets and millwork

Particle board containing urea-formaldehyde glue; porous surface materials (wood, solid polyester); numerous grout joints; recently applied lacquer, solvent varnish or acid-cured oil finish; recently applied plastic adhesive.

Solid wood, exterior plywood, or formaldehyde-free particle board; stone, nonporous composite, large ceramic tiles or plastic laminate; white glue; factory-cured finishes; all-natural, safe finishes.

Appliances

Kitchen

Gas cooktops and ovens; kitchens without exhaust fans; aluminum cookware.

Electric cooktops and ovens; ceramic cooktops; microwaves; convection ovens; stainless, glass and ceramic steamers and slow cookers; outside vented exhaust fans (see Ventilation).

Electrical

Lighting

Dependence on large fluorescent fixtures; dependence on cool white, or other poorly color balanced lamps; high-temperature lamp fixtures with plastic parts; poorly lit stairs and entries.

Halogen, tungsten and compact fluorescent lamps; daylight and full spectrum color balance (warm white lamps where appropriate); all metal and glass fixtures.

Electrical and magnetic field avoidance

Locating occupied rooms near service transformers, meters, main panels and large conductors or motors; locating televisions, computers, microwaves, and home office equipment near sleeping areas; sweep hand (motorized) clocks, small power supplies (e.g. battery chargers) and low-voltage lamps near beds; electric blankets; radiant electric panel heating near beds (above or below).

Separate utility rooms; places for televisions, computers and home offices chosen for distance from sleeping areas.

183

Heating and Air Conditioning

Convection and radiant heat

Unvented combustion heaters of any kind; fuel oil, coal- or wood-burning heaters with unsealed chimneys; very old or poorly maintained fireplaces or chimneys; chimneys discharging near windows or air intakes; high-temperature baseboard heaters; asbestos-covered hot water pipes.

Isolated or sealed combustion boilers; hot water, radiant floors or ceilings; hot water perimeter convectors; massive radiant heaters (e.g. European tile-oven).

Forced-air heat

Fuel oil or coal residues; old fuel oil, coal- or wood-burning furnaces; new, combustion or electric furnaces with high-temperature heat exchange; very old or poorly maintained chimneys; asbestos-covered furnace ducts; forced-air returns in contact with floor joists and stud cavities; ducts cast in concrete floors; oily residues in new ducts.

Isolated or sealed combustion boilers; heat pumps; hot water or heat pump fan-coil furnaces; sealed combustion chimneys; fully ducted forced-air returns; new ducts washed before installation; old ducts cleaned professionally.

Filtration

Minimum efficiency, conventional filters; filters with excessive restriction to air flow; old electronic filters (may produce excessive ozone); filters containing perfumes, antibacterial agents, oily tackifiers or quantities of adhesive (depending on sensitivities).

Medium-efficiency pleated filters; high-efficiency bag filters; carbon-treated fabric filters (for odor removal); bulk carbon, zeolite or other adsorbent odor-removal filters.

Cooling

Noisy, window-mounted units; compressors located in noise sensi-

Portable, water-cooled units; compressors located in landscaped and

AVOID	PREFERRED
tive areas; compressors exposed to excess sunlight; poor condensate drainage from evaporator coils.	screened areas; easily maintained evaporator condensate pans with a good slope to drain.

Water heating

Old combustion heaters; very old or poorly maintained chimneys.	Sealed combustion heaters; heat pump water heaters; electric water heaters; combined water heat/space heat systems.

Ventilation
Whole house

Large exhaust fans in a draft-sealed building with conventional chimneys; no ventilation system in a draft-sealed building in a cold climate; reliance on air leakage for supply air or combustion air in a cold climate; ventilation air intakes near chimneys, plumbing vents, dryer vents, allergenic plants, etc.; ventilation intakes ducted directly to furnace in very cold climates.	Supply air provided to each occupied room by furnace or ventilation ducts (cold climate); heat recovery ventilator (cold or hot climates); intake air slots in occupied rooms with whole house exhaust systems (moderate climate); intake air filtration in polluted locations; preheated ventilation air ducted to furnace in very cold climates.

Kitchen and bath exhaust

Noisy, ineffective fans; recirculating exhaust fans; excessive or restrictive exhaust ducts; corrodible ducts; moisture traps in ducts.	Quiet, high-capacity, multi-speed fans; smooth, direct duct runs; ducts sloped downward where moisture is expected.

Storage areas

Paint, cleaning supply, hobby supply and fuel storage connected to an occupied building.	Isolated storage areas; storage with a continuous exhaust fan; storage with outside vents.

Humidity control

Humidifiers using wicks or water reservoirs; humidifiers operated when relative humidity is above	Steam or ultrasonic humidifiers.

40%; humidifiers which deposit
water in air ducts.

Water Systems

Lead pipe or lead solder; PVC pipe
for heated water; untreated water
from surface sources or shallow
wells; drinking or showering with
heavily chlorinated water; drinking
or cooking with softened water (salt
flush softener systems).

Copper pipe with lead-free solder;
polyethylene or cross-linked polyethylene pipe; polybutylene pipe.

CHAPTER 10

Getting it Built

GETTING SPECIALIZED ADVICE

A healthy building renovation or construction project is different from a conventional project in several important ways. The emphasis in a healthy building project is on control of the environment, whereas in a conventional project, the emphasis is generally on time and cost. The case studies in this book indicate a range of possible strategies, while the 79 Best Healthy Building Solutions section shows some of the most successful details, systems and materials used in healthy buildings. Some of these healthy building elements are conventional approaches which have been refined, such as advanced moisture-proofing methods. Others, such as special materials selection and advanced heating and ventilating systems, are approaches that will be unusual to many, from the designer to the tradespeople who are working on site. In order for a healthy building project to be successful it is very important to establish at an early stage which approaches, systems and materials will be used. It is then essential to maintain communication throughout the project, to be sure it is built as intended. Without careful attention to detail and good communication, those involved in the construction are likely to default to their conventional practice, which may be exactly what was *not* wanted for the healthy building.

It is wise to begin your healthy building project by talking with someone who has done healthy building work before. This person may be an air quality consultant, an energy efficiency consultant with air quality experience, or an architect, engineer, building designer, interior designer or builder with specialized knowledge and experience. If this person cannot show evidence of specialized training and experience in healthy building, it's probably best to keep looking. In severe climates, those with training in energy efficiency are often the best qualified.

Consider using a specialized healthy building consultant who offers services such as predesign and design work, as well as specifications and project review. Consultants usually also offer environmental testing services where needed. They usually have training in architecture, building technology or interior design, but should also have some background in environmental sciences, such as health sciences, chemistry or physics. A healthy building consultant must have a detailed understanding of building science, ventilation and energy efficiency. There are national and regional environmental health associations which may be able to recommend a consultant to members. Some consultants may also be listed under Air Pollution Measurement in the telephone directory in major cities.

SELECTING AN ARCHITECT/DESIGNER AND CONTRACTOR

Remember that designing and constructing a healthy building is a challenge for all involved, and is often a test of organizational abilities. Even experienced designers and builders will usually have to do some research, rely on specialized consultants, and make unusual demands on tradespeople and suppliers to complete a healthy building project. For example, every item used on a jobsite, from the concrete in the foundation to the weatherstrip on the doors, may have to be scrutinized, depending on how rigorously nontoxic the building must be. Smoking is usually not permitted on site, and any substitution for materials or changes to details or systems will have to be carefully reviewed and approved.

Choosing an architect/designer and contractor for a healthy building should be a rigorous and thorough process. It is a good idea to check the candidate's references, and visit at least one of their completed projects, if possible. If you don't have any leads on possible consultants and builders, ask acquaintances who have built recently. It is also wise to check out a consultant's standing with his or her professional organization. Check to see if a contractor is registered with the local home warranty program and builder's association. Not all contractors participate in these programs or associations, particularly renovation contractors, but membership does provide some measure of consumer protection.

If a conventional bidding process will take place, there is one further caution. Contractors and their trades who are not familiar with the unusual requirements of a healthy building project are likely to balk when they sit down to price their work. In order to protect themselves from unknown factors, they may place high premiums in their bids for some healthy building features. It is wise for the owner or consultant to take extra care to provide as much detail as possible in the bid documents, and to speak with the contractors and trades before bidding. Have a personal meeting between the owners, contractor and consultants when turning over the bid documents, and encourage the contractor to phone with questions. Some flexibility in the contract is an advantage, for example cost allowances can be used for some items instead of bid prices. In this case a consultant will suggest a cost allowance amount for an item in a contract, such as floor coverings or cabinets, which may not have been decided or selected yet. Portions of the contract can also be "cost plus method" so that no extra is paid where no extra costs are incurred by the contractor. Contractors usually bill cost plus work at their cost, plus a small markup on materials, and a management fee. However, these methods increase uncertainty for the owner about final costs, and may be restricted if a mortgage holder is involved.

Some points which should be considered when choosing a designer and contractor are:

- As many details, materials and systems as possible should be selected and detailed during the design stages to reduce the number of expensive changes and delays during construction. Some healthy materials and system components take longer to select and receive, and this can cause scheduling problems which will halt construction.
- Specifications should be clearly spelled out, and the need for close adherence to them stressed. Any changes or substitutions to the specifications must be approved by the consultant and owner. It is not wise to use "equivalence"clauses in healthy building specifications which allow a supplier to substitute other materials or system components, because what is considered an equivalent by conventional standards may not be adequate for a healthy building.
- Though previous experience with healthy buildings may be hard to find, designers and builders with energy efficient building experience are often better prepared to understand the special construction techniques and exacting quality control required for a successful healthy building project.
- Remember that the designer and contractor are ultimately building specialists, not health professionals. They can only be expected to meet their respective obligations, and respond to the owner's requests. If there are specific health concerns involved, consult a health care professional.

BE YOUR OWN CONTRACTOR?

Many people consider acting as their own contractor on major remodeling or new construction projects. By hiring the demolition and excavation contractor, the framing contractor, the roofers, the electrician, and plumber and all of the other specialized trades directly, the owner hopes to save money and have more control. It is possible to save perhaps 10% to 15% of construction costs by managing your own project, and in view of the extra complexities involved in a healthy building there is merit in being in close control, but contracting is not for the faint-hearted or inexperienced. A good contractor has a great deal of experience with running a project, and knows how to coordinate trades and avoid delays and mistakes. They also know their people personally, and are familiar with building inspectors and local regulations. Someone who lacks practical experience and the necessary working relationships with tradespeople is very unlikely to be able to successfully and economically manage a complex project.

If you are an owner who has requested a healthy building, and will be hiring a consultant and contractor, you must be involved more than you would in a conventional project. You should expect to have several initial meetings with both, and be available for regular progress checks and decisions necessary during the process. Remember that even the best relationship between an owner and the designer and builder is likely to be strained before any building project is completed. This is even more likely when there are special requirements. Practicing patience and preparing well from the beginning is the best way to stay out of disputes and produce a successful project.

SUPERVISING CONSTRUCTION

If you are the contractor or specialized consultant for a healthy building project it is a good idea to begin construction with a meeting of as many of the people involved as possible. Even if it is necessary to pay the trades for a few hours of their time before they start work, this can pay for itself several times over in avoided problems. It is important to remember that tradespeople have the best knowledge of their specialty and wish to see the job done well. By discussing the healthy building practices and expectations from the beginning, and by going over each area of the work briefly in front of all of the trades, a good deal of helpful guidance can be gained from them. The questions and advice which come out of this meeting will often prevent future conflicts.

**NOTICE
CHEMICAL SENSITIVITY
ABSOLUTELY NO MATERIALS
ARE TO BE USED OR STORED
IN THIS BUILDING WITHOUT
PRIOR APPROVAL**

One of the most common and expensive problems in construction oc-curs when work which has been all or partly completed has to be removed due to late design changes or poor coordination of trades. The effect on the budget and the morale on site can be severe. For example, a concrete slab may have to be cut or demolished if the plumbing or wiring buried in it do not match the location of walls or cabinets. This can happen in any kind of construction if planning and communication are not adequate, or if changes are made too late. But in a healthy building, where healthy materi-als are emphasized, a completed or nearly completed installation may have to be removed if the material is wrong. Or finished walls and ceilings may have to be removed if unusual components of the heating and ventilation systems were not properly understood during rough installation.

Rigorous construction management is necessary to avoid contam-ination of construction for the envi-ronmentally hypersensitive.

Another important consideration is site cleanliness and organization. Especially on a healthy building project, it is well worth the time and effort to clean up every day after work in order to maintain safe and efficient work-ing conditions. Owners may do the cleanup themselves to save money.

MANAGING YOUR REMODEL

If you have a small remodeling project, it may be entirely appropriate to manage it yourself, if you have the right experience. Small projects are often

191

a nuisance to general contractors because their value is too low to justify the time they have to put in and the fees they must charge to manage it well. If you choose to manage your own small project, it is a good idea to observe all of the usual rules for contracting, only in a simplified form. Prepare clear and understandable drawings and notes, if not formal specifications. Never attempt anything more than a very simple replacement or repair project without drawings. These are the primary tool for communication in building design.

- Apply for permits as necessary. Check with your local municipal authority to determine when a building permit is required. Electrical, gas and plumbing permits are required for all work except simple repairs or replacement. These are usually the responsibility of the tradespeople.
- Interview potential trades and ask about their work. Try to find tradespeople through personal references or contacts, not through conventional advertising. Ask them what they will need in order to give you fixed prices for all or part of their work. But be aware that remodels are difficult to price exactly.
- Negotiate contract forms or letters of agreement with the trades. They will usually have their own forms, but these should be scrutinized closely for thoroughness and legal loopholes.
- Begin the work, and stay in close communication with anyone on the jobsite. Be there at least every second day.
- Do not prepay any contract amounts to trades, and limit your up-front investment to the purchase of any materials or equipment which you have agreed to buy yourself.
- Do not pay any invoices or progress amounts until you are sure that the work has been satisfactorily completed, and use a standard hold-back amount (often about 10%) on each invoice until at least 30 days after the total job is complete. Do not allow contractors access to credit or charge accounts which are in your name, and request a letter from the contractor before paying a large invoice, indicating that all amounts due to suppliers will be paid first before paying for the contractor's services.

Note: There are many good books on do-it-yourself contracting which contain contact sample forms and business and legal advice.

Do not expect a remodel to go as smoothly as a well-managed new construction project. One of the first maxims of remodeling is to expect trouble, especially in older buildings. It is inevitable that problems such as cracked foundations, rotted woodwork, framing that is not level or square, or inadequate insulation, wiring and plumbing will be found. You may even find asbestos, lead, urea-formaldehyde foam insulation, and other well-known health hazards which must be dealt with safely (sometimes requiring a specialized removal contractor).

If you are making large changes to an older building, such as adding new rooms or substantially restoring or remodeling, remember that building standards have changed substantially in the past 80 years, and the local authorities are likely to require that much of the remaining building be brought up to current building safety standards. This might involve expensive additions such as fire separations and sprinklers, earthquake bracing and additional insulation, even in single-family homes in some areas.

Finally, don't expect fixed prices for all items on a remodeling project. And don't use square foot costs for estimating renovation costs. They are just too unreliable. Some remodeling costs more per square foot than new construction. The only trades which are likely to be able to give reliable fixed prices are electrical, plumbing and heating, and then only when the system is to be substantially replaced. For the foundations, framing and finishing trades, it is often difficult to predict how much time and work will be involved. Consequently they may insist on doing all or part of their work on an hourly basis.

POST-CONSTRUCTION CLEANUP

One way to save money is to do at least some of the cleanup yourself. Remember that all construction debris should be removed from the building the same day it is produced. It can be stored outside, or inside in a sealed container. Also remember that no debris should be left in the building's cavities. No solvents, paints, oils, grease, liquid fuels or other similar substances should be stored in the building, and make sure that no cleaning of paint equipment is done in the building, and that no spray applications are done in remodels or occupied buildings.

Dust Removal

- *Coarse dust removal:* Brush any ceilings, walls, doors or other surfaces which have not been freshly painted with a soft brush to pick up coarse materials and dislodge clinging dust. Lightly sweep floors, counters, appliance tops and other objects to pick up accumulated debris.
- *Vacuuming:* If drywall, plaster or insulation has been handled

indoors, vacuum only with a built-in vacuum vented outside the living space, or with a portable HEPA vacuum, available from rental stores or purchased from a vacuum supplier. These vacuums have special fine filters, and are also known as "allergy vacuums." First vacuum walls and ceilings using a soft brush on the vacuum head. Vacuum the floors last, using a power brush if available.

- *Duct cleaning* (in remodels): If the furnace system has not been cleaned for two years or more, or if the furnace was used to heat part of the house during construction, have the ducts cleaned by a commercial service. Services which use an air hose to dislodge dust may be more effective.

- *Surface wiping:* Go over all smooth wall surfaces, doors and wood-work with a clean, damp cotton cloth dipped in a solution of 4 tablespoons of white vinegar to 1 gallon (60 ml to 4 liters) warm water. Rewet the cloth regularly and wring it out well. Discard the cloth or launder it when it shows signs of soiling, and change the water and vinegar regularly. There is no need to rinse the vinegar solution off. Do not attempt to wipe textured ceilings and delicate wallpapers or other surfaces which are not scrub resistant.

- *Floors:* First scrub spots and spills on wood, ceramic or linoleum floors with a sponge or gentle pot scrubber as necessary. Use only a mild solution of soap, or a cleaner known to be safe for occupants. Then mop the entire floor area with a new sponge mop or string mop using 4 tablespoons of white vinegar to 1 gallon (60 ml to 4 liters) warm water. Rewet and wring out the mop regularly, and change the water when it becomes murky. There is no need to rinse the vinegar solution off. Do not use vinegar on unsealed stone or ceramic floors, or cement grout.

  Cracks in wood floors or grout joints in tile floors may require a dampened scrub brush to remove dust and dirt. Carpet cleaning is a special case and should only be done with specialized healthy building advice.

- *Bathroom and kitchen wet surfaces:* Make a solution of 3 tablespoons (45 ml) of borax crystals (the standard laundry product) to a quart (liter) of boiling water. Stir it and let it cool overnight, then filter through a coffee filter or paper towel. Put this in a hand pump sprayer (e.g. an atomizer used for house plants) and spray it on wall tile, counter tops, shower doors and around the edge of baths and showers. It can also be used to help prevent mildew damage where windows sweat by spraying it on frames and sills. Do not rinse it off, but repeat the application as often as twice a week in the bathroom. In a remodel, if tile and tubs and showers are badly stained with mildew, clean them first. Standard hydrogen peroxide and an old toothbrush usually works. More stubborn stains can be removed with a dilute bleach solution, but do not do this while a sensitive person is at home. At least 12 hours of airing out is recommended after bleach cleaning. Only use prepared tile cleaners which are known to be safe for the person. Badly stained silicone caulking will have to be replaced while the sensitive person is away.

- *Glass cleaning indoors:* First scrub or scrape stubborn spots or stickers off glass. A mild washing soda solution can be helpful if needed (see Cleaning stubborn or greasy areas, below). Then wipe glass with a soft absorbent cloth and solution of equal parts water and white vinegar. No need to rinse. Polish glass with a dry cloth.
- *Final filtration and ventilation:* After floor cleaning is complete, begin operating the furnace and any other air circulation, filtration or ventilation equipment to reduce suspended dust. Operate it continuously for at least 24 hours before moving in. Check that the filters are not overloaded.
- *Cleaning stubborn or greasy areas* (in remodels): For greasy areas such as around kitchen ranges, and for stubborn spots on floors or counters, make a solution of 4 tablespoons (60 ml) of washing soda (sodium carbonate, the standard laundry product) in a quart (liter) of hot water. Apply it with a sponge or pot scrubber, not with a brush because it splatters. Always wear gloves and protect your eyes when handling washing soda. It is very caustic to the skin.
- *Exterior scrubbing:* Deck surfaces, concrete, siding, patios and stairs which have signs of mildew and algae growth can be power-washed, or scrubbed with a brush and soapy warm water. A little bleach can be added also. If soap is used, rinse after. Do not power-wash siding or use a hose on it without testing to be certain that it will not deteriorate or leak water into the walls.

Ozone Treatment

Ozone treatment may be used in enclosed spaces for sterilizing fungus (mildew) contaminated areas and reducing mildew odor and residual smoke odor. It may also be used to reduce odor from fresh paint, vinyl, upholstery materials, etc., and in new automobile interiors. A high-potency generator capable of at least 400 milligram of ozone per hour is recommended for rooms up to about 300 square feet (30 square meters), if the air exchange rate is minimal. For larger areas, or unenclosed spaces, plastic tents are recommended to concentrate the ozone in the treatment area. Exposure times of about two hours should be used on a trial basis, judging by odor reduction if more treatment is necessary.

Be cautious if soft plastic materials such as vinyl upholstery covers or wallpaper are present. These may be damaged by excessive ozone treatment.

People, pets or house plants should not be in the rooms while concentrated ozone treatment is in progress. People who are not hypersensitive, and have no respiratory problems, such as asthma or emphysema, may be in the vicinity (in the building, but not in the treatment area), but should vacate the area if burning nose or eyes occurs.

Airing out rooms for about one hour after ozone treatment is sufficient to make them safe to reinhabit. Ozone has a very short life, but the by-products of ozone treatment may result in unusual odors for some time afterwards. These odors are a nuisance only and are not hazardous.

Recommended Cleaning Products

- Baking soda
- Unscented soap
- Dilute vinegar
- Borax in water
- Dilute hydrogen peroxide
- Washing soda in water (sodium carbonate)

79 Best Healthy Building Solutions

Foundations, Drainage and Termite Protection

Preventing ground moisture and soil gas entry. Non-toxic, mechanical termite protection.

Structural Systems

Durable structures, minimizing use of (or isolating) glue-bonded materials.

Siding and Roofing

Durable weather protection minimizing use of plastics, asphalt and sealants.

Roof and Crawl Space Venting

Preventing trapped moisture and reducing summer overheating.

Draft Sealing and Insulation

Controlling air migration in insulated cavities to prevent contamination and damage.

Noise Control

Preventing noise entry and transfer between rooms.

Non-Toxic Finish Details

Durable and easily maintained interior surfaces, minimizing use of sealants, paints and plastics.

Sunlight and Daylight

Climate adapted use of free energy.

Heating, Ventilating and Water Treatment

Maintaining comfort and controlling air quality through appropriate heating, cooling, ventilating and filtering methods. Improving water quality by filtration and non-toxic sterilization.

Foundation Drainage System, Dry Region

A perimeter perforated pipe covered with gravel collects water and leads it away from the foundation. It must be located below the basement slab level. Rain water and groundwater should only be combined where heavy rainfall does not occur, and where soil conditions are very porous. Always carry the drain line away to lower ground, or to a storm drain with a backflow prevention device to reduce flooding risk.

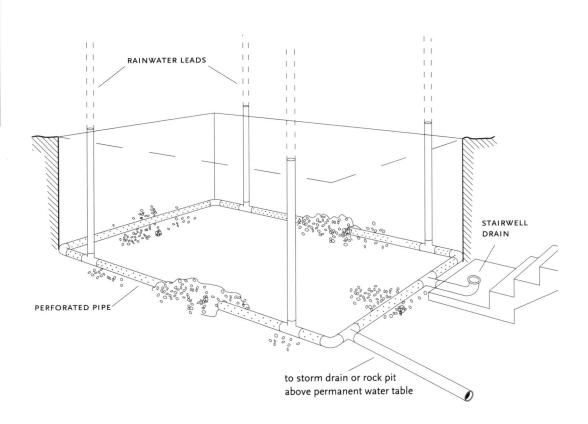

RAINWATER LEADS

STAIRWELL DRAIN

PERFORATED PIPE

to storm drain or rock pit above permanent water table

Foundation Drainage System, Dry Areas

In dryer climates, or on very well-drained sites, the rainwater system can be combined with the foundation drainage. A drainage filter material should be placed over the gravel to prevent sediment from plugging it. This system shows the foundation insulated from the outside for a cold climate. The insulation must be covered with cement plaster or cement board where it projects above the ground. Exterior insulation not recommended in termite zones.

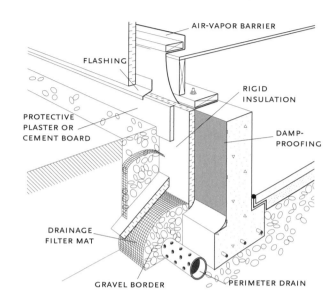

AIR-VAPOR BARRIER

FLASHING

RIGID INSULATION

PROTECTIVE PLASTER OR CEMENT BOARD

DAMP-PROOFING

DRAINAGE FILTER MAT

GRAVEL BORDER

PERIMETER DRAIN

Foundation Drainage System, Wet Areas

In wet climates, or on poorly drained sites (such as those with heavy clay soils), the rainwater system should be separated from the foundation drainage. The rainwater system is made from solid pipe, and the foundation drains from perforated pipe. This system shows the foundation insulated from the outside for a cold climate. The insulation must be covered with cement plaster or cement board where it projects above the ground. Exterior insulation is not recommended in termite zones.

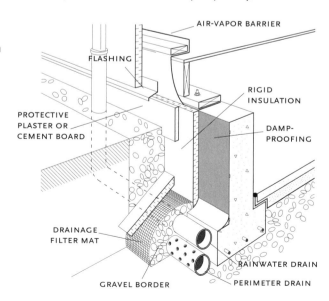

AIR-VAPOR BARRIER

FLASHING

RIGID INSULATION

PROTECTIVE PLASTER OR CEMENT BOARD

DAMP-PROOFING

DRAINAGE FILTER MAT

RAINWATER DRAIN

GRAVEL BORDER

PERIMETER DRAIN

Insulated Basement Slab, Mild to Cold Climates

Keeping the basement slab warm is important for moisture control and comfort. The basement slab can be insulated with a rigid insulation board installed below. (The insulation board should be rated for use under a slab.) In a mild climate the edge of the slab can be insulated from the outside. The moisture barrier should be brought up to the slab edge and caulked.

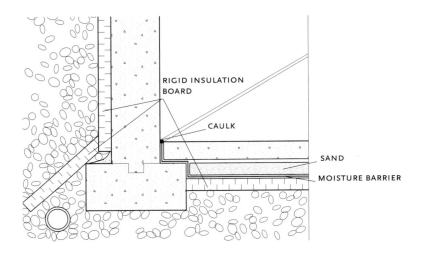

Insulated Slab Edge/Heated Slab

The slab edge should be carefully insulated, especially in colder regions. The insulation can extend horizontally for two feet beyond the building edge. *Note*: Termite shields should be used in termite areas. A heated slab edge is difficult to insulate adequately in very cold climates.

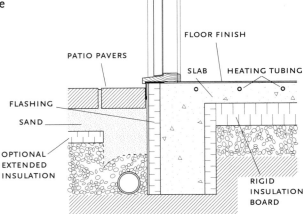

Insulated Basement Wall and Slab (can be retrofitted)

Basement slabs and walls should be insulated in cold or humid regions to prevent moisture problems and improve comfort. Rigid insulation board can be used if rated for this purpose. Sealing joints around trims and preventing wallboard from contacting the concrete is important for moisture control.

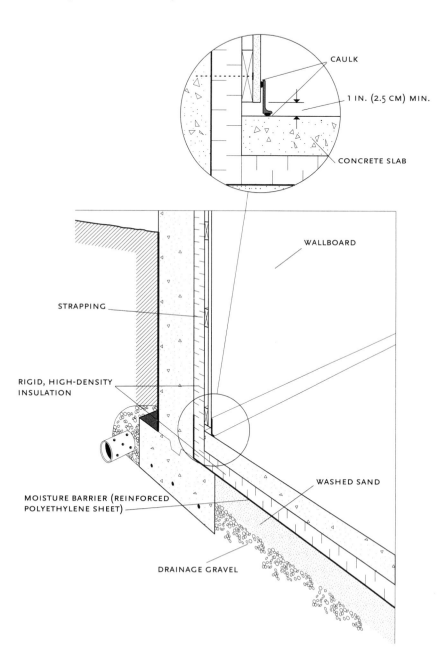

CAULK

1 IN. (2.5 CM) MIN.

CONCRETE SLAB

WALLBOARD

STRAPPING

RIGID, HIGH-DENSITY INSULATION

MOISTURE BARRIER (REINFORCED POLYETHYLENE SHEET)

WASHED SAND

DRAINAGE GRAVEL

Patching Basement Cracks

All cracks should be thoroughly sealed to prevent soil gas, insects and moisture from entering. Flexible caulking should be used between the slab and wall, and in any small cracks. Expanding cement patching mortar is better for larger cracks. Cracks should be enlarged and cleaved before filling.

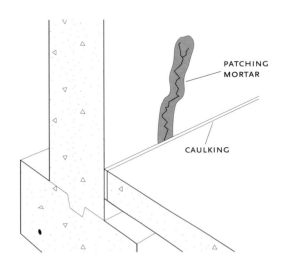

PATCHING
MORTAR

CAULKING

Soil Gas Prevention at Floor Drain

Special floor drain fittings are available which will securely seal the drain against soil gas entry.

(ball floats when water enters)

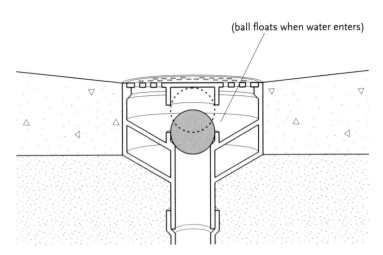

Soil Gas Venting System Below Slab

In regions with high risk of soil gases, a system of perforated pipes placed in gravel and connected to a continuous exhaust fan may be used to reduce gas entry.

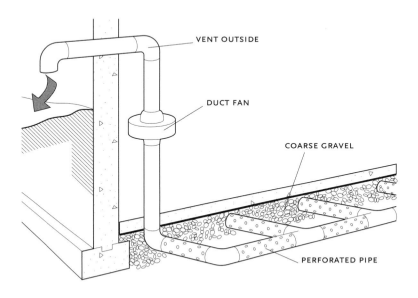

VENT OUTSIDE

DUCT FAN

COARSE GRAVEL

PERFORATED PIPE

Sealing Sump Against Soil Gases

A basement sump should be securely sealed using a cover with a gasket. It should be vented to the outside of the building.

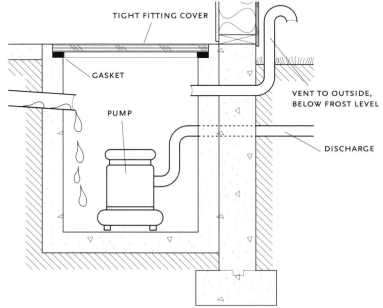

TIGHT FITTING COVER

GASKET

PUMP

VENT TO OUTSIDE, BELOW FROST LEVEL

DISCHARGE

203

Sheet Metal Termite Shields at Perimeter Foundation

Concrete foundations and pipes entering the building from the soil should be shielded approximately 12 inches (30 centimeters) from the ground to prevent termites from reaching the wood. The termites may attempt to build tubes to climb up to the wood, so these areas must be inspected periodically, and tubes removed. A barrier zone of sand or diatomaceous earth will help prevent termites from climbing the foundation.

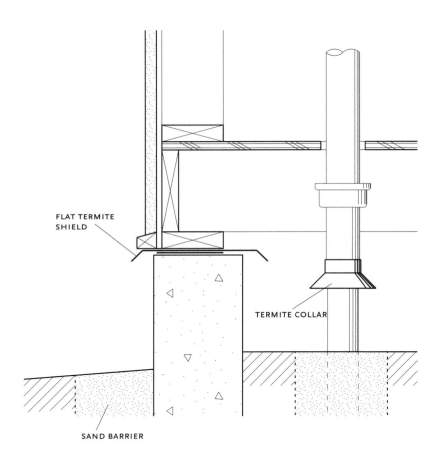

FLAT TERMITE SHIELD

TERMITE COLLAR

SAND BARRIER

Termite and Rodent Barrier at Chimney Base in Crawl Space

All masonry and post supports in a crawl space should be fitted with termite barriers in termite-prone regions to prevent them from reaching the wood framing. This barrier is inserted into the masonry and projects out about 3 inches (7.5 centimeters). The underside of joists should also be covered with metal screen, plywood or waterproof gypsum to prevent insects and rodents from entering the house through the crawl space.

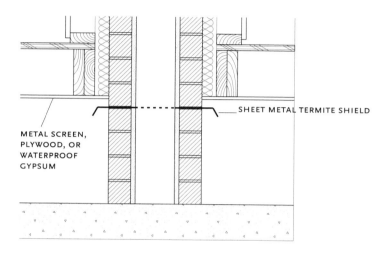

METAL SCREEN, PLYWOOD, OR WATERPROOF GYPSUM

SHEET METAL TERMITE SHIELD

Termite Shield Key

In termite-infested areas, a sheet metal key should be installed at the joints between stem walls, to prevent termites from entering through the cracks which often develop at these points.

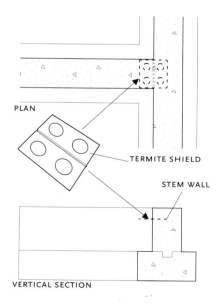

PLAN

TERMITE SHIELD

STEM WALL

VERTICAL SECTION

Sheet Metal Termite Shields at Porch or Deck

Concrete foundations and pipes entering the building from the soil should be shielded approximately 12 inches (30 centimeters) from the ground to prevent termites from reaching the wood. The termites may attempt to build tubes to climb up to the wood, so these areas must be inspected periodically, and tubes removed. A barrier zone of sand or diatomaceous earth will help prevent termites from climbing the foundation.

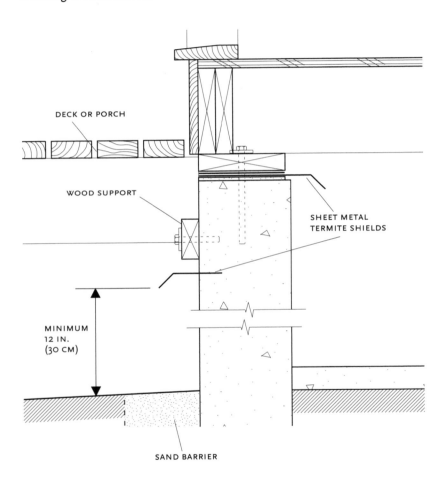

DECK OR PORCH

WOOD SUPPORT

SHEET METAL TERMITE SHIELDS

MINIMUM 12 IN. (30 CM)

SAND BARRIER

Sheet Metal Termite Shield at
Interior Load-bearing Wall on Concrete Slab

Termites may enter the house through small cracks which often develop in concrete as it cures and settles, particularly at load-bearing walls. A sheet metal termite shield can be cast into the concrete under the wall to prevent entry. The cast-in shield will "bridge" any cracks which occur, preventing termite entry from surrounding soil.

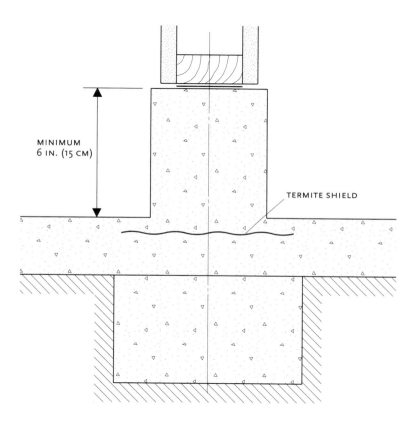

MINIMUM
6 IN. (15 CM)

TERMITE SHIELD

Various Sheet Metal Termite Components

Sheet metal termite shield components are standard for many types of wood plate, post and sill construction. There are inside corners, outside corners and connector pieces.

A) 2-SIDED COMPONENTS FOR CRAWL SPACE CONSTRUCTION

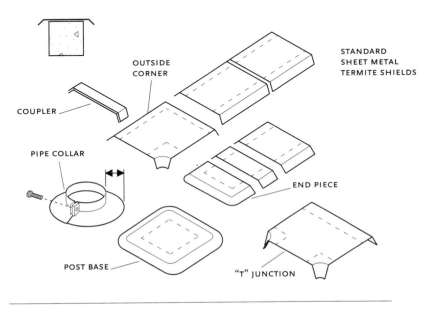

OUTSIDE CORNER

STANDARD SHEET METAL TERMITE SHIELDS

COUPLER

PIPE COLLAR

END PIECE

POST BASE

"T" JUNCTION

B) 1-SIDED COMPONENTS, SLAB OR BASEMENT CONSTRUCTION

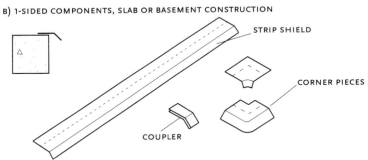

STRIP SHIELD

CORNER PIECES

COUPLER

Exterior Insulation Sheathing with Wall Brace System

It is possible to eliminate much of the structural wall sheathing in some buildings by using a steel brace system. This is not only resource efficient, but eliminates glue and wood products. Rigid insulation board can then be used behind the siding to improve insulation and weather resistance if required. Seek engineering advice, especially in windy or earthquake zones.

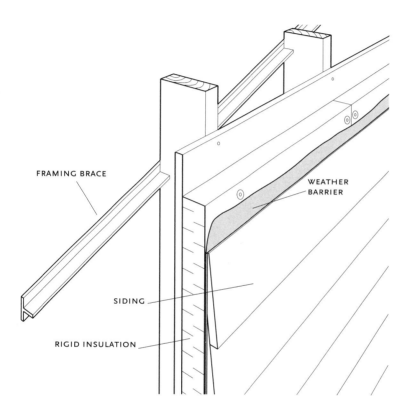

FRAMING BRACE

WEATHER
BARRIER

SIDING

RIGID INSULATION

Brick Clad Wall with Steel Framing

Brick may be used over wood or steel framing, using an air cavity and providing weep holes in the brick mortar. This is among the most durable and weather-resistant finishes. The bricks must be tied to the structure with metal straps. Stainless-steel straps are best for corrosion resistance. The brick support system must be engineered, particularly in earthquake zones. If metal framing is used, exterior insulation board should be used to improve the building insulation. This system can completely eliminate wood, plastic and paint from the exterior walls.

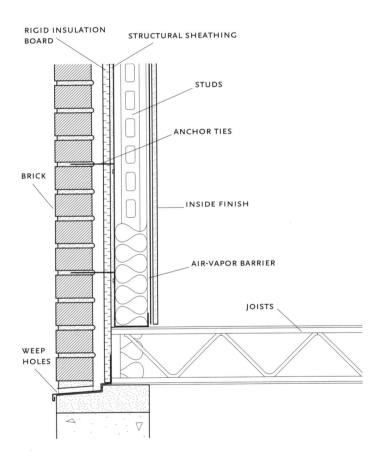

RIGID INSULATION BOARD

STRUCTURAL SHEATHING

STUDS

ANCHOR TIES

BRICK

INSIDE FINISH

AIR-VAPOR BARRIER

JOISTS

WEEP HOLES

Steel Framing on Concrete Block Foundation

Steel framing can be supported directly on a perimeter wall. Concrete block may be used if the soil depth doesn't exceed approximately 4 feet (1.2 meters). The basement or crawl space can be insulated with a non–load-bearing wall, allowing for an airspace which will prevent moisture transfer. Steel framing of outside walls should always be insulated with an exterior insulation board. This system can eliminate all wood, plastic and paint from the wall. In a very mild climate the insulated interior wall may be eliminated.

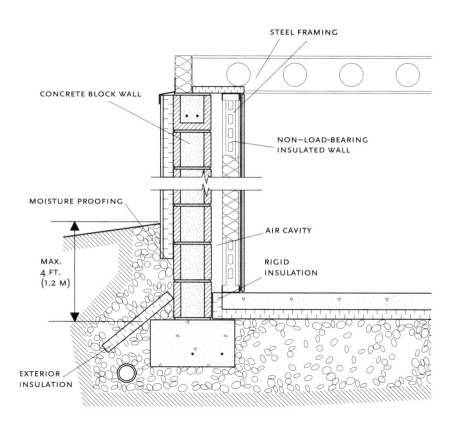

STEEL FRAMING

CONCRETE BLOCK WALL

NON–LOAD-BEARING INSULATED WALL

MOISTURE PROOFING

AIR CAVITY

MAX. 4 FT. (1.2 M)

RIGID INSULATION

EXTERIOR INSULATION

Open Web Floor Joist System

Open web floor joists are available which are substantially more stable and reliable than solid wood and have no glue in them. They also allow ducts, pipes and wires to run without drilling. Special blocking and installation details are required, however. Seek engineering advice.

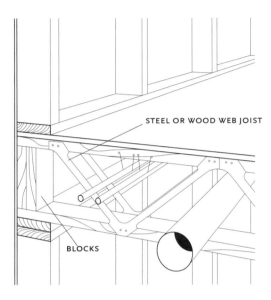

STEEL OR WOOD WEB JOIST

BLOCKS

Concrete Suspended Slab System

Concrete slab construction can be used for upper floor construction in buildings, usually with masonry or concrete supporting walls. These have the advantages of sound and fire resistance, durability, thermal mass and minimal dust-collecting surfaces. A corrugated steel sheet is usually used for a form, and then a ceiling suspended from it later, though the ceiling is optional.

REINFORCED
SUSPENDED SLAB

STEEL DECK FORM

CEILING
FURRING
STRIPS

WIRE TIES

CEILING

Air-sealing Solid Wood Subfloor and Sheathing

Older homes were built with solid boards (usually shiplapped). Some still use shiplap today to avoid glue-bonded materials. It is important to seal the subfloor edge outside the rim joist, and to place a gasket under the sill plate to reduce air leakage. When renovating a building this is best done from outside. It can be partially done from inside using caulking and expanding foam.

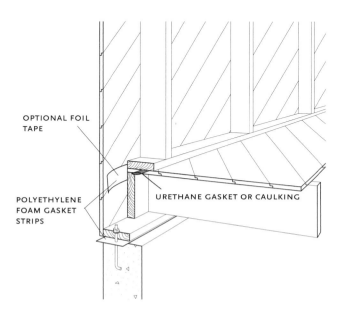

OPTIONAL FOIL TAPE

POLYETHYLENE FOAM GASKET STRIPS

URETHANE GASKET OR CAULKING

Raised Heel Roof Trusses for Improved Insulation And Venting

In cold or hot (air conditioning required) climates the roof insulation is especially important at the wall and soffit. A raised heel truss is built up with a block at this point to allow thicker insulation and unobstructed flow of roof ventilation. An insulation stop prevents insulation from blocking the ventilation path.

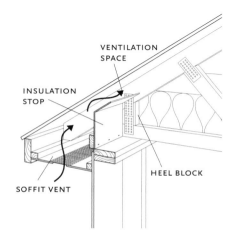

VENTILATION SPACE

INSULATION STOP

SOFFIT VENT

HEEL BLOCK

All-steel Floor and Roof Framing

Building with steel avoids all wood and wood products in the building. Termite protection is therefore unnecessary. Load-bearing and non–load-bearing (lightweight) steel components are standard for building types where combustible materials are not allowed by code. They are fastened with screws and clips, and can be cut with a special saw or snips. Insulating a steel building is difficult, however, because steel conducts heat. Special details and advice are needed for very cold or hot (air conditioning required) climates. Double stud walls can be used for more insulation. Seek engineering advice.

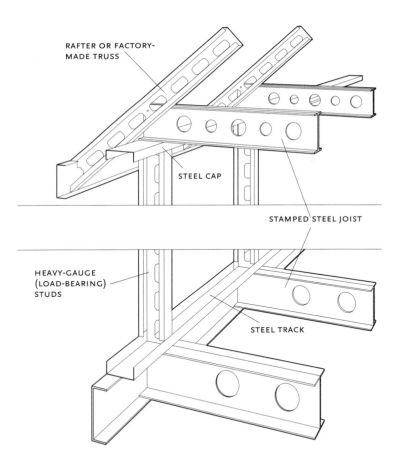

RAFTER OR FACTORY-MADE TRUSS

STEEL CAP

STAMPED STEEL JOIST

HEAVY-GAUGE (LOAD-BEARING) STUDS

STEEL TRACK

Steel Framed Roof System

A roof system can be built using light steel trusses, purlins and steel roofing. It is highly durable and contains no wood, adhesive or asphalt. A weather barrier sheet or thin insulating board should be used under the roofing to prevent condensation from dripping into the cavity. Ventilation of the cavity is also critically important to prevent corrosion. In colder regions, insulated sheathing board should be used on the ceiling to improve insulation.

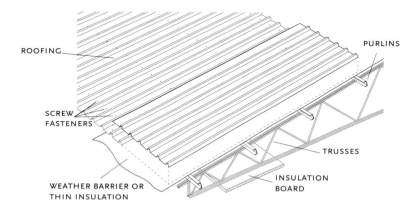

ROOFING

PURLINS

SCREW FASTENERS

TRUSSES

WEATHER BARRIER OR THIN INSULATION

INSULATION BOARD

Steel Stud, Non–Load-bearing Partitions

Steel studs can be used for partition framing in a wood-framed building to reduce the amount of wood used indoors. Steel studs are also unlikely to warp and buckle as they dry, a common problem with wood framing. If load-bearing wood walls are expected to shrink, a wood plate can also be used for the steel-framed wall, or a steel track can be used with clearance for settling. Seek engineering advice.

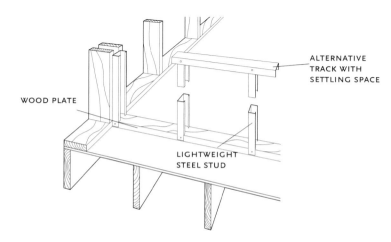

ALTERNATIVE TRACK WITH SETTLING SPACE

WOOD PLATE

LIGHTWEIGHT STEEL STUD

Exterior Insulation and Stucco

Stucco may be placed directly on mesh mounted on exterior insulation board. The structural sheathing or framing should be protected with a moisture-impermeable layer to prevent leaks from damaging the structure. *Note*: This system should not be relied upon to prevent moisture from entering in extremely weather-exposed situations. It needs substantial weather shelter, except in very dry climates.

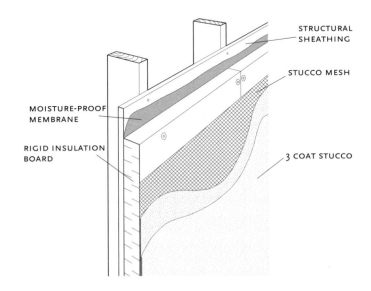

STRUCTURAL SHEATHING

STUCCO MESH

MOISTURE-PROOF MEMBRANE

RIGID INSULATION BOARD

3 COAT STUCCO

Flashing of Shingle Roofs

A shingled roof must have full flashings at the eaves, ridges and valleys to achieve its full lifespan and reliability. In wet climates, a strip of pure zinc metal placed just below the ridge will reduce moss growth on the shingles and extend their life. Metal or fiber-cement shingles are the most durable types.

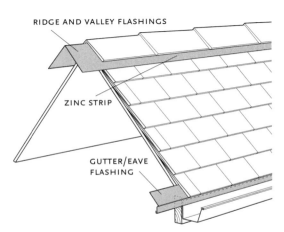

RIDGE AND VALLEY FLASHINGS

ZINC STRIP

GUTTER/EAVE FLASHING

Torch-On Roof Membrane

Where flat or shallow pitched roofs are necessary, a factory-made membrane of modified asphalt and crushed slate can be installed by heating the underside and seams with a large torch. The membrane is durable, and avoids the mess and pollution of hot tar roofing methods. It has far less odor than rubber membranes.

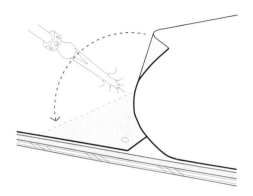

Inverted Flat Roof System

Where flat roofs are necessary, an "inverted system" uses a waterproof membrane on the roof deck, covered by rigid insulation board which is protected from weather and prevented from floating by gravel ballast. The membrane lasts longer and insulation performs better under the ballast. A drainage mat is necessary to prevent the drainage paths from plugging with roof debris.

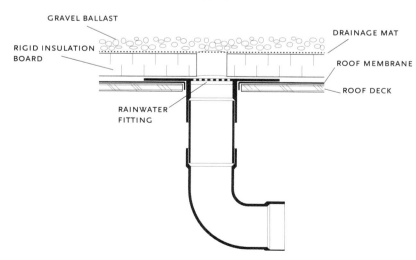

Venting Attic Spaces

In winter, heated air which leaks into the attic must be allowed to escape immediately to avoid moisture damage. First the warm air leakage paths should be minimized, then an inlet path and escape path for outdoor air should be provided.

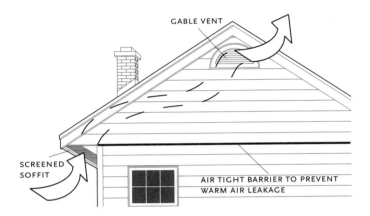

Venting Roof Spaces

In vaulted, insulated ceiling construction, a small, continuous air space must be left above the insulation. This should be fed by a screened soffit vent, and vented at the ridge by a screened ridge vent, or by several roof vent fittings.

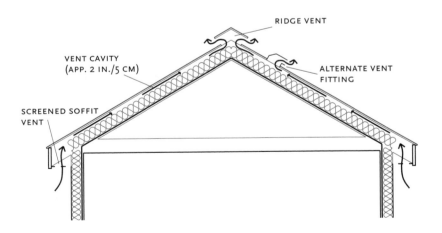

218

Venting Attic Spaces

Any insulated rooms in the attic must be designed to allow air to escape between the insulation and the roof.

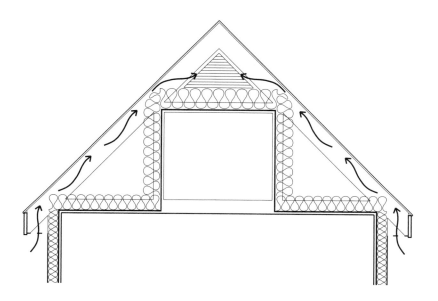

Ventilating an Unheated Crawl Space

When the floor is insulated, the crawl area must be fitted with screened vents to allow moisture in the space to dry. One square foot of vent is adequate for about 200 sq. ft. of crawl space (0.5%). In very cold regions, the vents can be partially closed in winter. Note that the insulation encloses any ducts or pipes, and the crawl floor has a moisture barrier and thin concrete slab to keep it dry and clean.

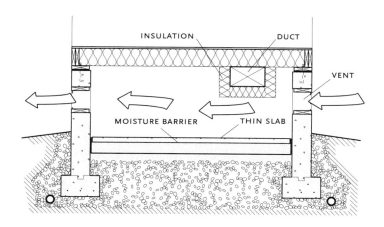

219

Insulating and Vapor Sealing a Bay Window

The insulation and vapor barrier must be fully extended into the bay window. In a cold climate the floor and roof section must be well insulated. Any heating ducts must be inside the insulation, and air-sealed where they enter the bay. Note that the air vapor barrier in the floor stays on the inside of the insulation.

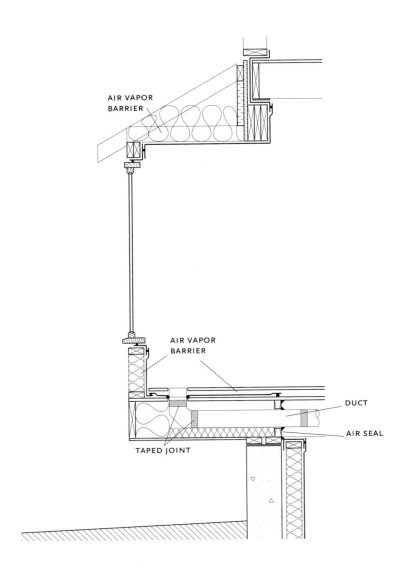

AIR VAPOR
BARRIER

AIR VAPOR
BARRIER

DUCT

AIR SEAL

TAPED JOINT

Rain Screen Wall Construction

A rain screen wall will prevent water damage to the building in exposures where strong wind-driven rain occurs. It will also provide better insulation to minimize indoor condensation as well as excellent soundproofing from outdoor noise. The wall is first sheathed with an insulating board or, in warm climates, with just a sealed weather barrier. This surface is then divided into compartments using straps (horizontal or vertical) to create an air space of at least 1/2 inch (1.2 centimeters). The siding is then applied to the straps. The air compartment is vented at the bottom, and closed at the corners and top. The compartments equalize air pressure, preventing rain from seeping into the wall. Horizontal straps need gaps in them to allow drainage.

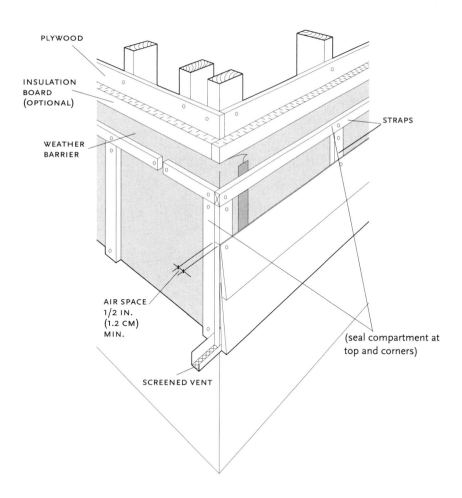

PLYWOOD

INSULATION
BOARD
(OPTIONAL)

WEATHER
BARRIER

STRAPS

AIR SPACE
1/2 IN.
(1.2 CM)
MIN.

(seal compartment at
top and corners)

SCREENED VENT

Warm Air Leakage, Cold Weather

In cold weather, moist, warm indoor air which leaks into insulated cavities through openings at windows, door jambs, electrical outlets and plumbing penetrations is likely to condense on cold spots, leaving moisture damage and mold growth.

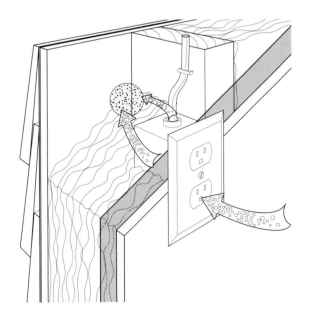

Warm Infiltration, Warm Weather

In warm or windy weather, contaminated air carrying molds, odors and dust is likely to enter the house through these same leakage paths. *Note*: This same phenomenon can occur in reverse in warm climates during air conditioning.

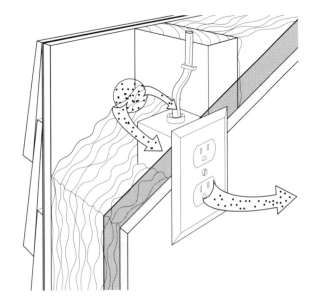

Sealing a Door Opening to the Air Vapor Barrier

Air leakage at the door frame is a common cause of discomfort, and can cause excessive drying of wood components. A polyethylene sheet should be wrapped around the frame and taped to the air vapor barrier on the inside and the weather barrier sheathing on the outside. Any gaps left after mounting the door jamb should be filled with expanding foam.

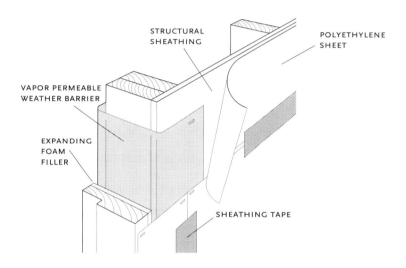

STRUCTURAL
SHEATHING

POLYETHYLENE
SHEET

VAPOR PERMEABLE
WEATHER BARRIER

EXPANDING
FOAM
FILLER

SHEATHING TAPE

Sealing Air Vapor Barrier to Electrical Outlet

In insulated walls, a polyethylene boot is installed behind electrical boxes and taped to the air vapor barrier when it is installed. The wires should be caulked where they pierce the boot. Special molded boxes with gasketed flanges are also available.

Note: This is the solution to the problems illustrated on the opposite page.

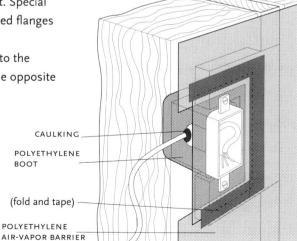

CAULKING

POLYETHYLENE
BOOT

(fold and tape)

POLYETHYLENE
AIR-VAPOR BARRIER

Sealing Air Vapor Barrier at Window Opening

Air leakage at the window frame is a common cause of discomfort, and may cause the wood components to warp and the windows to stick. Joining the air vapor barrier to the exterior weather barrier with tape and filling gaps with expanding foam will minimize leakage.

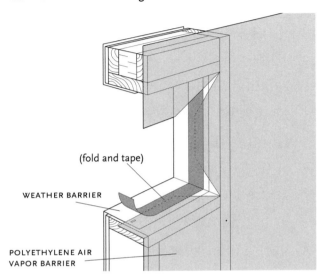

(fold and tape)

WEATHER BARRIER

POLYETHYLENE AIR
VAPOR BARRIER

Sealing Air Vapor Barrier to Window Frame

As an alternative to sealing the vapor barrier to the weather barrier, a polyethylene strip installed during framing can be joined to the air vapor barrier of the wall with tape. Any gaps left *after* mounting the window should be filled with expanding foam.

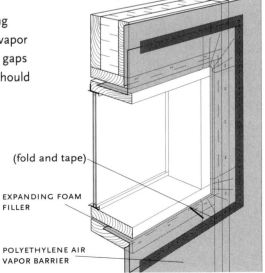

(fold and tape)

EXPANDING FOAM
FILLER

POLYETHYLENE AIR
VAPOR BARRIER

Sealing Wall Air Vapor Barrier at Partition

A partition wall joined to an insulated wall must provide continuity for the air vapor barrier. During framing, the end stud of the partition can be wrapped with polyethylene which is later stapled and taped to the air vapor barrier of the wall. Note that the rim joist of the floor framing can also be joined this way.

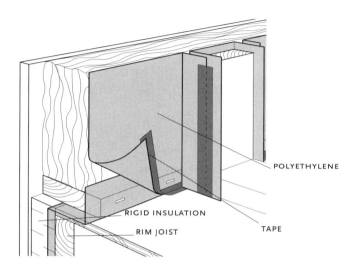

POLYETHYLENE

RIGID INSULATION

RIM JOIST

TAPE

Sealing Ceiling Air Vapor Barrier at Partition

A partition wall joined to an insulated ceiling must provide continuity for the air vapor barrier. During framing the top plate of the partition can be wrapped with polyethylene which is later stapled and taped to the air vapor barrier of the ceiling.

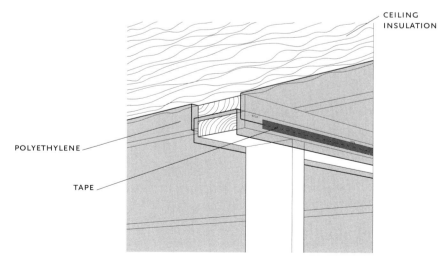

CEILING INSULATION

POLYETHYLENE

TAPE

225

Preventing Noise Transmission Between Spaces

Doors and windows separated as much as possible (see Plan B) reduce sound transmission. Extending the wall up through a suspended ceiling and sealing the base in a sound-absorbing floor finish will reduce sound transfer between rooms (see Section D).

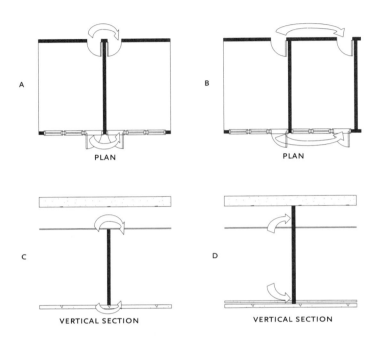

A — PLAN

B — PLAN

C — VERTICAL SECTION

D — VERTICAL SECTION

Tile Floor with Acoustic Isolation

A tile floor transmits impact sound easily. Placing tile on 2-inch (5 centimeters) lightweight concrete and suspending a double gypsum board ceiling on resilient bar will reduce sound transmission. The cavity should be filled with insulation.

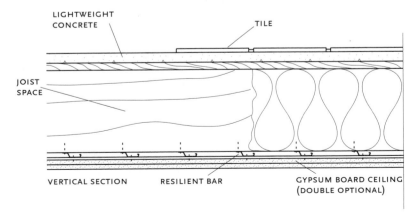

LIGHTWEIGHT CONCRETE

TILE

JOIST SPACE

VERTICAL SECTION

RESILIENT BAR

GYPSUM BOARD CEILING (DOUBLE OPTIONAL)

Isolated Wall Framing System

Wall framing can be isolated by staggering framing on plates which are 2 inches (5 centimeters) wider than the studs. The cavity space should be filled with insulation. Double gypsum board walls, or plaster on an insulating board will also reduce sound transmission.

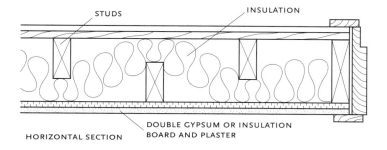

STUDS INSULATION

DOUBLE GYPSUM OR INSULATION
BOARD AND PLASTER

HORIZONTAL SECTION

Isolated Ceiling Framing System

A separate ceiling support system can be used to reduce the transfer of sound. Independent framing is installed between the main joists to support only the ceiling. The space between is filled with insulation, and often an acoustic underlay, such as fiber gypsum board, is used under the finish flooring to further reduce impact noise. Where floors are strong enough, 2 inches (5 centimeters) of lightweight concrete can also be used as a flooring underlay. Double gypsum board ceilings also reduce noise.

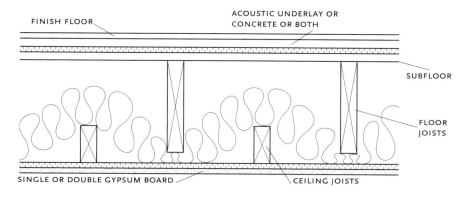

FINISH FLOOR ACOUSTIC UNDERLAY OR
CONCRETE OR BOTH

SUBFLOOR

FLOOR
JOISTS

SINGLE OR DOUBLE GYPSUM BOARD CEILING JOISTS

VERTICAL SECTION

Resilient Ceiling Suspension

Another way to isolate sound through gypsum and plaster ceilings is to suspend them on a special steel strip called a resilient bar, available from gypsum board suppliers. The bar is slightly springy and will reduce sound transmission through the framing.

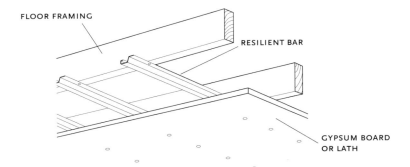

FLOOR FRAMING

RESILIENT BAR

GYPSUM BOARD
OR LATH

Resilient Wall Suspension

Walls can also be suspended on resilient bars. The bars are screwed to the studs, and the gypsum board screwed to the floating portion of the bar. Solid backing strips are usually needed at the bottom to support baseboard trims.

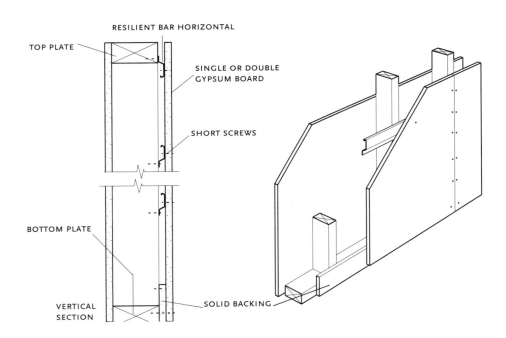

RESILIENT BAR HORIZONTAL

TOP PLATE

SINGLE OR DOUBLE
GYPSUM BOARD

SHORT SCREWS

BOTTOM PLATE

SOLID BACKING

VERTICAL
SECTION

Resilient Bar Detail

The resilient bar is screwed to the framing on one side. The gypsum board is then screwed to the floating part of the bar with short screws to prevent them going through to the framing.

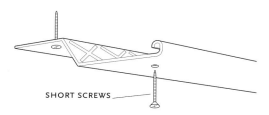

SHORT SCREWS

Isolating Plumbing Noise and Plastic Odors

Plastic plumbing is noisy and has a styrene or vinyl odor which bothers some people. After installation the drains can be wrapped with heavy aluminum foil and sealed with foil tape to reduce the odor. The holes for the pipes must be oversize to reduce noise transmission into framing. Caulking the openings will help to reduce noise and odors from plastic. Cast-iron or copper drains are a better option, but are expensive.

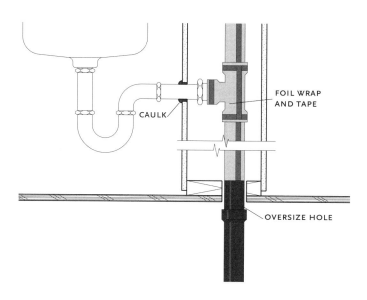

FOIL WRAP AND TAPE

CAULK

OVERSIZE HOLE

Inside Insulation with Plaster Finish

Wood or steel framing can also be insulated from the inside with rigid insulation board, forming a base for plaster. The insulation board is screwed to the framing and covered with metal or plastic lath to receive the plaster. A vapor barrier must be provided if the insulation board is vapor permeable. *Note:* Exterior plaster mixtures may not be appropriate inside the healthy house due to chemical additives.

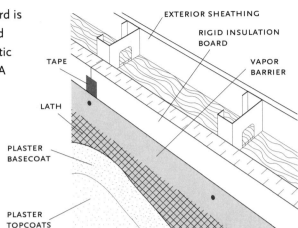

Adding Interior Insulation and Finish

An older home with walls in poor condition can be repaired from the inside while upgrading the insulation. The electrical outlets can be extended with standard extension rings. The window and door frames will also have to be extended and have trims reinstalled. The new system must be tightly air sealed to prevent moisture leakage into cavities. A vapor barrier is usually not necessary if old plaster and paint are left intact.

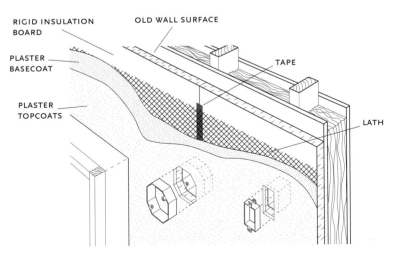

Plaster Details for Baseboards

Traditional plastering methods are sometimes used for healthy buildings to avoid the paper, fillers, sanding and paints necessary for gypsum board. Plaster work is a fine art, but can still be done by some plaster and stucco contractors. At the base of the wall, one or two wood strips called "grounds" are placed on the framing to guide the plasterer, and as a mount for the final base and trim boards. Plaster may be placed on metal lath, gypsum board or masonry surfaces.

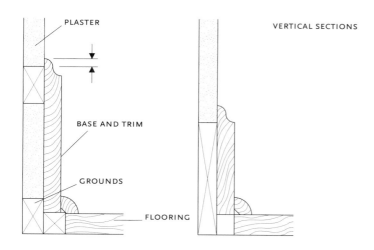

PLASTER

VERTICAL SECTIONS

BASE AND TRIM

GROUNDS

FLOORING

Ceramic or Irregular Flagstone Floor

Sealing the floor to the wall is important for dust control and to prevent mop water from seeping into cracks. A smooth tile floor can be easily sealed to a baseboard with a safe caulking, such as silicone or siliconized acrylic. Irregular floors, such as handmade tile or flagstone, should be fitted with a ceramic cove tile.

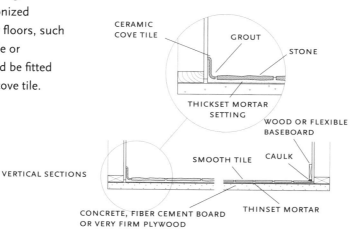

CERAMIC
COVE TILE

GROUT

STONE

THICKSET MORTAR
SETTING

WOOD OR FLEXIBLE
BASEBOARD

VERTICAL SECTIONS

SMOOTH TILE

CAULK

CONCRETE, FIBER CEMENT BOARD
OR VERY FIRM PLYWOOD

THINSET MORTAR

Plaster Trim Details

Traditional plaster work can be used at door and window openings in conjunction with tile, wood or precast plaster veneer trims (available from specialty suppliers).

A) Tiled opening on plaster base. The tile is applied to plaster with thinset mortar. Either a wood casing or bullnosed tile may be used for the edge trim against the plaster.

B) Wood or precast plaster trimmed opening. The material is nailed or screwed directly to the framing. A wood or plaster trim may be used for the edge trim against the plaster.

C) All wood trimmed opening. Standard wood casings can be used in the opening and against the plaster by nailing them to the "ground."

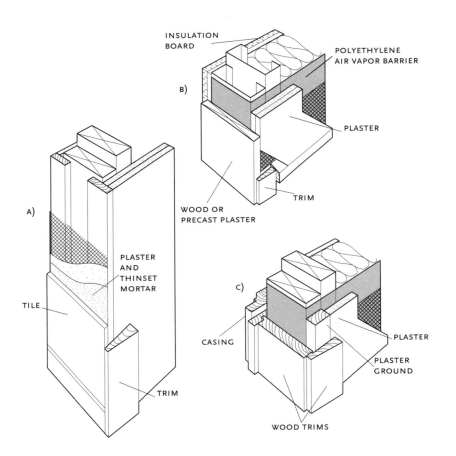

Wood Floor over Concrete

One method of anchoring wood flooring to concrete without glue is to use a steel channel and clip system. The concrete is covered with a moisture barrier, if necessary, and the channels are anchored with concrete nails or screws and shields. A clip system then holds the wood flooring.

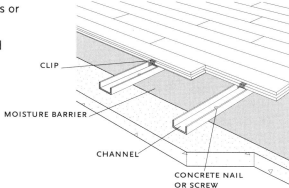

CLIP

MOISTURE BARRIER

CHANNEL

CONCRETE NAIL
OR SCREW

Low-pollution Cabinet Construction

Cabinets made with conventional particle boards, glues and some finishes are a source of indoor pollution. A new cabinet which is closed for long periods will collect the emitted gases and release them when opened. Cabinets may be made from solid or formaldehyde-free particle board to reduce the pollution load. Metal and glass components may also be used. Water-based carpenter's glue is a safer alternative for assembly, and factory-applied and -cured lacquers (solvent or water based) are safer finishes. See Materials Selection in chapter 9. Building cabinets off site and aging them before delivery will help to reduce dust and gas exposure on site.

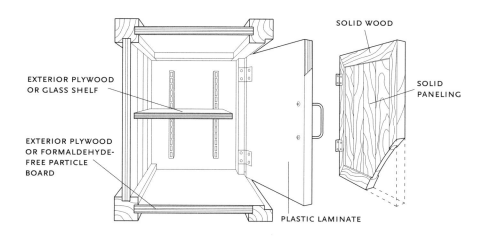

SOLID WOOD

SOLID
PANELING

EXTERIOR PLYWOOD
OR GLASS SHELF

EXTERIOR PLYWOOD
OR FORMALDEHYDE-
FREE PARTICLE
BOARD

PLASTIC LAMINATE

Furniture Construction

Most new furniture is made with treated fabrics, plastic foams, glues and pressed wood products which release irritating gases for long periods. New furniture should be made with low-toxicity and easily cleanable materials. As furniture ages it collects dust and begins to deteriorate, making it a source of dust. Washable covers and barrier cloth (a specially woven fabric which encloses dust) inner covers will make cleaning more effective.

Some environmentally sensitive people find that older, solid wood furniture can be restored with safe, pre-washed fabrics and fillings to produce an acceptable result. Others have custom work done in carefully self-tested safe materials. Care must also be taken to avoid contamination with dust and odors while work is in the shop or in storage.

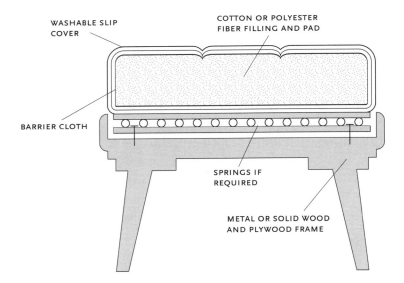

WASHABLE SLIP COVER

COTTON OR POLYESTER FIBER FILLING AND PAD

BARRIER CLOTH

SPRINGS IF REQUIRED

METAL OR SOLID WOOD AND PLYWOOD FRAME

Using Solar Heat and Shade

Careful roof design and window location will allow sun to enter from fall to spring when the sun's altitude is low, while shading in summer when it is high. In cold, sunny climates, some additional thermal mass such as a concrete or brick wall, or multiple layers of gypsum will help store heat. The opportunities for solar heating and shading are very specific to the climate and the building design. They can be calculated by an energy expert for optimum design.

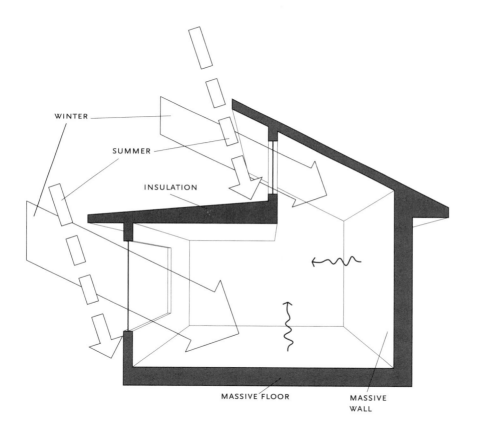

WINTER

SUMMER

INSULATION

MASSIVE FLOOR

MASSIVE WALL

Add-on Greenhouse Window

A greenhouse window can be added to a room with an east or south exposure to greatly improve light and sun. A west exposure is not recommended in most situations. Inside surfaces should be glass, metal or ceramic to prevent moisture and sunlight damage. Those very sensitive to molds may find some dry-climate houseplants acceptable, particularly if the potting soil is kept covered with a layer of fresh sand and activated carbon to reduce release of mold and odors.

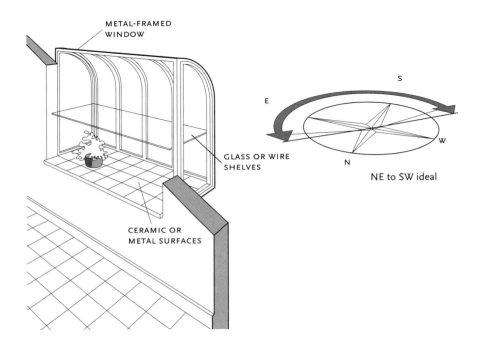

METAL-FRAMED
WINDOW

GLASS OR WIRE
SHELVES

CERAMIC OR
METAL SURFACES

S

E

W

N

NE to SW ideal

Heating, Ventilation and Filtration System

The fan-coil furnace provides healthy heating from a hot water source or heat pump, excellent filtration and, if required, cooling. The fan can be run continuously at low speed. A separate ventilator delivers outdoor air into the fan coil, after preheating it through an energy recovery core in colder climates. The ventilator extracts humid, stale air from the bath and kitchen. Note that the return air to the fan coil is located high in the rooms to capture warmer air for comfort and energy benefits.

Note: Always locate ventilator intake well away from garages, pollen producing plants, sewer vents, gas meters, garbage collection areas or any other source of pollution.

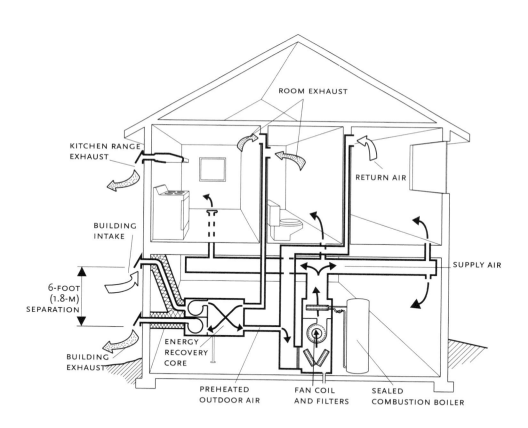

ROOM EXHAUST

KITCHEN RANGE EXHAUST

RETURN AIR

BUILDING INTAKE

SUPPLY AIR

6-FOOT (1.8-M) SEPARATION

BUILDING EXHAUST

ENERGY RECOVERY CORE

PREHEATED OUTDOOR AIR

FAN COIL AND FILTERS

SEALED COMBUSTION BOILER

A Fan-coil Heating and Cooling Unit

A good-quality fan coil can provide gentle, healthy heat from a hot water source, while offering excellent filtration. It also provides ventilation air, and cooling if required. The low-temperature heating does not burn dust, and produces much less odor than a conventional furnace.

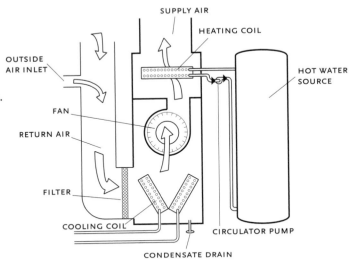

SUPPLY AIR
HEATING COIL
OUTSIDE AIR INLET
HOT WATER SOURCE
FAN
RETURN AIR
FILTER
COOLING COIL
CIRCULATOR PUMP
CONDENSATE DRAIN

A Sealed Combustion Boiler

A sealed combustion, gas-fired boiler or water heater, also called a "condensing unit," can provide both hot water and heating for the home. The risk of flue gas leaking into the home is extremely small. Sealed combustion heaters and boilers are over 90% efficient and therefore cost 20% to 30% less to operate than conventional burners. A drain is required for the condensed water produced by the burner.

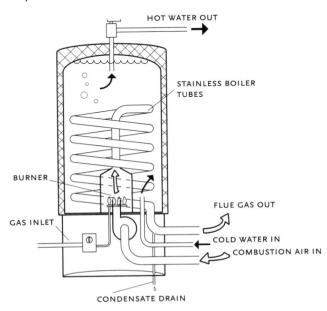

HOT WATER OUT
STAINLESS BOILER TUBES
BURNER
FLUE GAS OUT
GAS INLET
COLD WATER IN
COMBUSTION AIR IN
CONDENSATE DRAIN

Typical Boxed Joist Space and Fully Ducted Joist Space

A) Return air ducts formed by enclosing wood floor joists are very prone to collecting dust and debris, and harboring stale odors and microorganisms. They also draw air randomly from many leaks, and are nearly impossible to clean thoroughly.

B) A fully sheet metal–lined return duct avoids most of the problems of boxed joists. However, wiring and plumbing runs through the space will be more restricted.

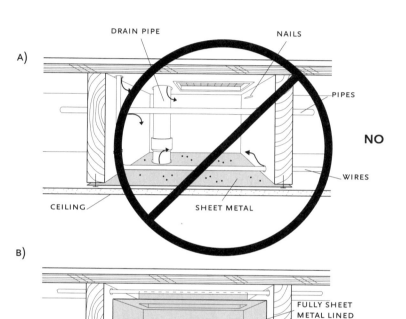

Ventilation System for Radiant Heat or Convectors

When radiant heat or convectors are chosen for heat, there will be little ducting in the home and no air filtration. Excellent air quality can still be achieved through dust control and ventilation. In a cold climate a ventilator should supply air to each bedroom and living space, and exhaust stale, humid air from the kitchen and bath. An energy recovery unit can preheat the incoming air by extracting heat from the exhaust air. Intake and exhaust ducts should be insulated to prevent condensation.

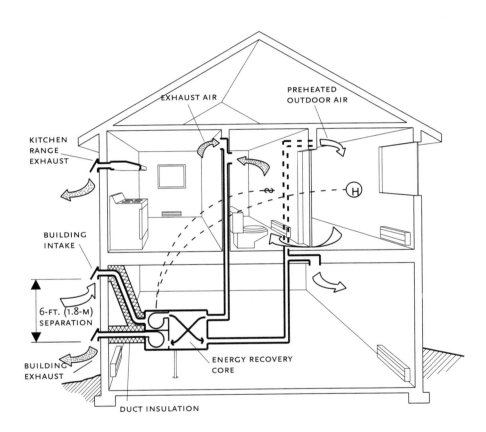

EXHAUST AIR

PREHEATED OUTDOOR AIR

KITCHEN RANGE EXHAUST

BUILDING INTAKE

6-FT. (1.8-M) SEPARATION

BUILDING EXHAUST

ENERGY RECOVERY CORE

DUCT INSULATION

Heated Basement Floor with Tile Finish

Hot water radiant heat can be used over a new or existing basement slab. The tubing should be placed on rigid insulation board and embedded in concrete. Tile can then be set on the concrete with thick or thinset mortar or the concrete can be colored and sealed as a final floor. The slab edge and walls should be insulated and finished with gypsum board or plaster. The heating thermostat should measure the floor temperature, not the air temperature.

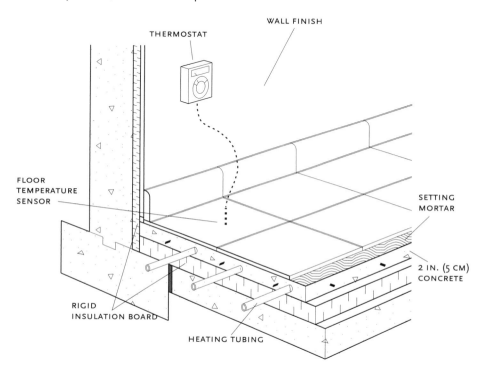

THERMOSTAT

WALL FINISH

FLOOR TEMPERATURE SENSOR

SETTING MORTAR

2 IN. (5 CM) CONCRETE

RIGID INSULATION BOARD

HEATING TUBING

Hot Water Radiant Ceiling Heat

Hot water radiant heat has health advantages, but often it is difficult to install in a floor, or some people may not want a warm floor. Radiant heating can be achieved by installing pipes in the ceiling and embedding them in plaster. First, rigid insulation board is installed and covered with foil to direct the heat downward. Then pipes are hung on loose fitting clips, and the spaces between them filled with gypsum board strips. Lath and plaster can then be installed over the strips. Extra insulation above the pipes is required for cold climates if installed against an insulated ceiling.

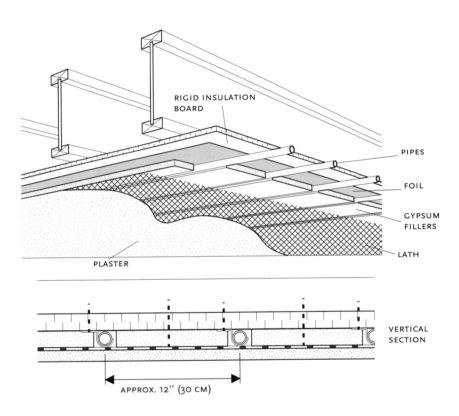

RIGID INSULATION BOARD

PIPES

FOIL

GYPSUM FILLERS

LATH

PLASTER

VERTICAL SECTION

APPROX. 12" (30 CM)

Low-Temperature Convector

Where electric heating is chosen, a low-temperature, liquid-filled unit has air quality benefits. A sealed electric coil at the bottom heats a liquid which flows through a finned convector, heating the room air which passes over it. The surface temperature remains much lower than conventional electric heaters, so dust is not cooked and odors are less. All convectors require regular vacuum cleaning of the fins.

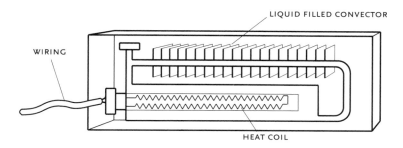

LIQUID FILLED CONVECTOR

WIRING

HEAT COIL

Portable, Low-Temperature Radiator

Healthy heat can be added to a single room by using a low-temperature, portable electric radiator. The unit contains a large, liquid-filled heat exchanger which is heated by a sealed electric coil at the bottom. These are very safe, due to low surface temperatures, and more easily cleaned than convectors. Be certain that the wiring is adequate for these units, and do not use extension cords.

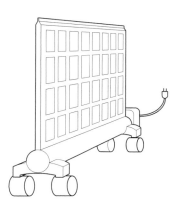

Heat Pump Furnace System

Where electricity is the heating fuel a heat pump furnace is a healthy option due to its low-temperature operation and air filtration ability. It is two to four times more efficient than direct electric heating. The outdoor unit contains a compressor which extracts heat from the air (in mild climates) or the soil or groundwater (in colder climates) using a refrigeration cycle. The heat is transferred to a low-temperature fan coil indoors, providing air quality benefits similar to a hot water furnace. High-performance filtration is easily included, and the cycle may be reversed for cooling in summer. Equipment must be professionally installed and maintained to prevent refrigerant leaks.

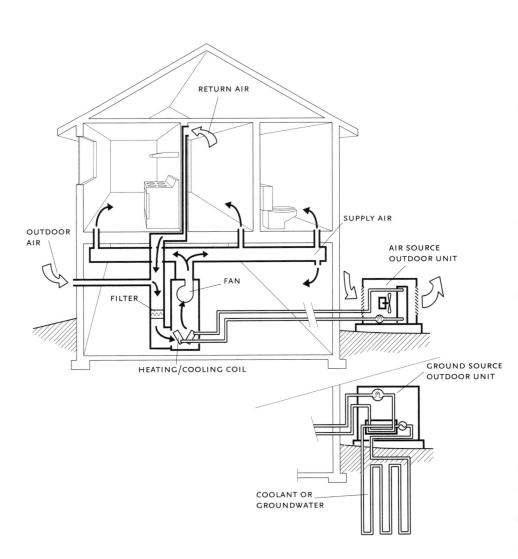

RETURN AIR

SUPPLY AIR

OUTDOOR AIR

AIR SOURCE OUTDOOR UNIT

FAN

FILTER

HEATING/COOLING COIL

GROUND SOURCE OUTDOOR UNIT

COOLANT OR GROUNDWATER

Split System Air Conditioner

One way to add air conditioning to a room or a suite is to use a split system. This type has an evaporator unit with a fan mounted permanently on a wall. The condensor and compressor are mounted outdoors, on the ground or roof. These are very quiet and efficient, though the outdoor unit makes some noise. All air conditioning tends to reduce indoor humidity.

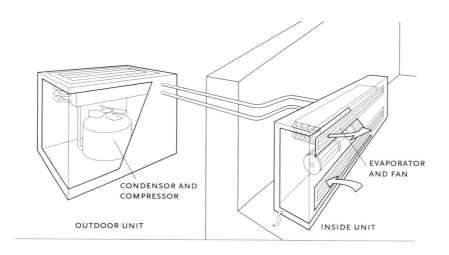

CONDENSOR AND
COMPRESSOR

OUTDOOR UNIT

EVAPORATOR
AND FAN

INSIDE UNIT

Portable Air Conditioner, Water Cooled

In some climates, a portable air conditioner may be needed periodically, especially in an older home without central air conditioning. One type of portable unit uses a water reservoir to cool the condensor, then discharges humid, warm air outdoors through a flexible duct. This type is more efficient and quieter than a window-mounted unit.

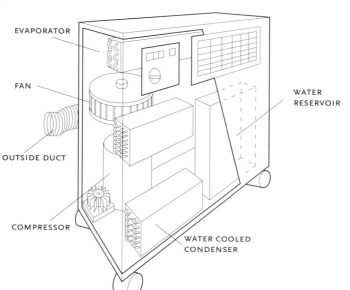

EVAPORATOR

FAN

OUTSIDE DUCT

COMPRESSOR

WATER
RESERVOIR

WATER COOLED
CONDENSER

Air Filter Efficiency

There are three test methods used for air filters. The Atmospheric Dust Spot Method should be the reference for medium- and high-performance filters such as furnace filter upgrades. 20% to 40% efficiency is a good range for add-on filters. For special air handlers with better fans, bag filters up to about 85% efficiency can be used. Electronic filters offer the highest efficiency for typical furnaces and air handlers without excessive restriction. HEPA (High-Efficiency Particulate Arrestance) filters are usually used only in special air cleaners such as portable units or bypass units.

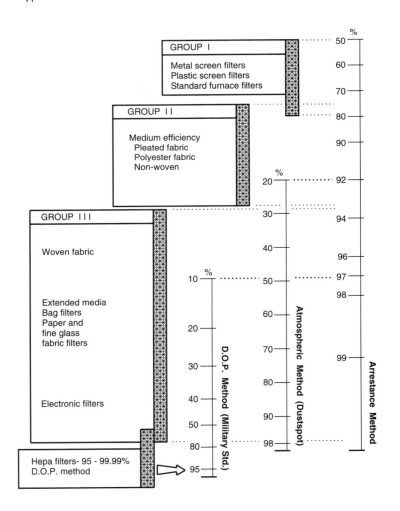

Pleated Medium-efficiency Filter

This filter type is made from a folded fabric, usually polyester. It is a good upgrade where a conventional furnace must be used. It is several times more efficient than a standard furnace filter, yet provides no extra resistance because of the extended surface area. It is best to use at least a 2- to 4-inch thick unit (5 to 10 centimeters), the thicker the better.

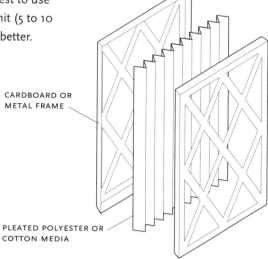

CARDBOARD OR
METAL FRAME

PLEATED POLYESTER OR
COTTON MEDIA

Bag Filter

A bag filter can be used in an air handler with a powerful fan. These offer high efficiency and extended life, but require extra space. With normal use they generally need replacement only after one or two years. They are made of polyester or glass fiber fabric. Some bag filters contain objectionable adhesive and perfumes. A wet-laid, glass paper filter is another option which usually contains less adhesive and fits in a similar space.

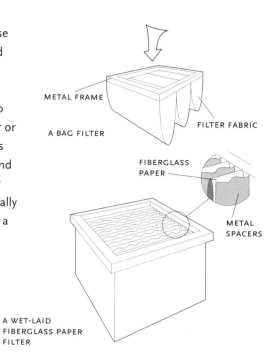

METAL FRAME

A BAG FILTER

FILTER FABRIC

FIBERGLASS
PAPER

METAL
SPACERS

A WET-LAID
FIBERGLASS PAPER
FILTER

Scrubbing Outdoor Air

The outdoor air supply may need to be scrubbed of particles and odors in some locations before it is brought in to the building. Outdoor air from a supply fan can be passed through a series of filters before entering the fan coil or furnace. The filters must be as effective as possible, because they only contact the air once. They must also not be too restrictive for the supply fan.

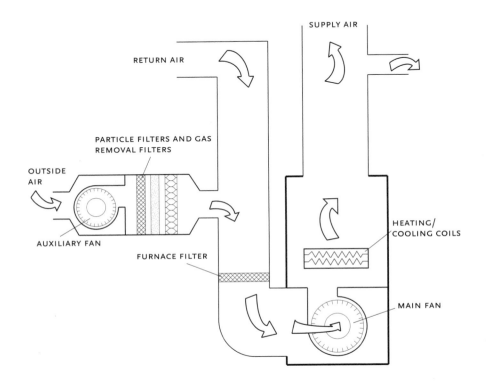

Bypassing Furnace Filter

Very high-performance filters, such as HEPA filters and carbon scrubbers, can be installed in a fan-coil furnace, or even a conventional furnace. The filters are placed in a separate housing and part of the return air is diverted through them, then back to the furnace. Often a separate booster fan is required, interlocked to the furnace fan control. Consult a specialized heating contractor for advice.

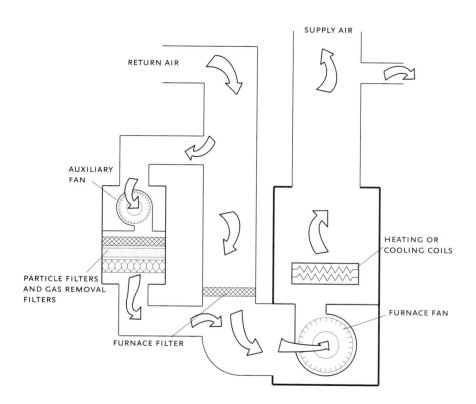

RETURN AIR

SUPPLY AIR

AUXILIARY FAN

PARTICLE FILTERS AND GAS REMOVAL FILTERS

FURNACE FILTER

HEATING OR COOLING COILS

FURNACE FAN

Appendix A

COMMON QUESTIONS AND ANSWERS ABOUT HEALTHY BUILDINGS

Can a sick building make someone chronically ill if the person has never been allergic or sensitive before?

Yes, definitely. Many types of exposures are sensitizing, that is, they cause a person with normal health to eventually become reactive. A common example is exposure to fungus particles and high dust levels, especially irritating wood dust. Many people with no previous history of allergy as children have become allergic as adults. This is due to the fact that our immune system response can increase with prolonged exposure, to the point where the immune response itself becomes a cause of discomfort and distress.

Is radon in homes really as risky as was thought a few years ago?

Perhaps not, but don't dismiss it. Radon is thought to increase lung cancer risk, especially among smokers. It is also thought to produce some cancers among nonsmokers. The question is, how much risk is there, and at what radon level? The answer to this is uncertain.

The action level (level above which steps to reduce exposure are recommended) chosen in the United States for radon reduction in homes is 4 pCi/l (4 picocuries per liter), which was determined by large statistical studies of uranium miners. Action levels in Canada and Europe are much higher, about 20 pCi/l. Since then, at least two major studies of populations with elevated radon levels in homes have failed to find a strong link with cancer rates above those in homes without radon. However, this does not mean that radon doesn't have a role in cancer. It does! It just means that the chosen action levels may not be appropriate, or that the wrong questions have been asked in the studies. Radon has never been viewed as a short-term risk. If it is going to increase cancer risk, it will do so over a period of decades. It is still wise to pay attention to it, but perhaps we can relax a little more about those homes which are close to the lower action level of 4 pCi/l.

Do indoor plants really remove volatile organic compounds such as formaldehyde and toluene from air?

Only indirectly. This has been widely misunderstood since early work done by Bill Wolverton at NASA was publicized. Plants themselves do not absorb and break down organic vapors through their respiration; however, the soil organisms around the roots of a healthy plant do. The problem is that gases move very slowly into the soil, so the effect is very small. Wolverton actually developed the idea of the living air filter, which uses a fan to force air through a soil bed containing activated carbon and plants. This is much more effective because the air is brought into contact with the subsoil. This can also be done with an "air washer," which dissolves air pollutants in water and then distributes them to plant roots.

The first priority when cleaning indoor air is to remove the source of indoor pollutants, rather than relying solely on an air treatment method. Of course there are many other compelling reasons to have plants indoors. They contribute a great deal to our quality of life and the beauty around us. They offer color, growth, seasonal change and fragrance. They also humidify. But those who are sensitive to molds should be cautious. Plants that prefer a dryer soil should be chosen, and the soil surface covered with a fresh layer of sand and activated carbon to reduce mold emissions release.

Who is affected by indoor pollution?

Everyone is affected to some extent. Just as about 25% of people are considered "allergic" to environmental conditions in the usual sense (that is, they suffer from hay fever, asthma or other well-recognized disorders triggered by plant materials or animal dander), there are also people who are sensitive to chemical exposure. It is hard to say how many are affected because of individual variation, but it is likely that most of us are sensitive to some environmental incitants. Healthy buildings are not only for environmentally sensitive people, they also play an important role in prevention.

What can be done in a rented building?

There are a surprising number of things a tenant can do to make a rental healthier, and not all are expensive. Some building problems will have to be repaired by the owner, for example, water damage, leaky chimneys, faulty heating and air conditioning, and smoke and fire damage. So make sure to select a rented accommodation carefully, and find a responsible owner who has maintained it well. Does the building have adequate ventilation? A kitchen and bathroom fan and one opening window per room is a minimum. Is the air outside acceptable to you? Is it relatively free from street pollution, pollens and other problems? Does it have a dust problem, a soiled carpet, dampness or mildew? Is the noise level acceptable to you? Does it have enough daylight? Does it have a furnace with dirty ducts and bad smelling air? (Many prefer a hot water heating system.) How is the water quality?

If a building is chosen in a clean location, with older plaster and hardwood finishes, and hardwood, metal, glass and cotton furniture and area rugs are used, it will be a good basis for a healthy building. Cleaning and polishing with simple soaps, vinegar, baking soda and other healthy cleansers instead of hazardous chemical products containing chlorine, ammonia and solvents will also help. A large-capacity, portable air filter and some bright lighting will improve an imperfect situation. Many people also buy a portable water purifier which, along with air filters and lights, can be taken when they move. The tenant can also take responsibility for painting, and select a safe paint, asking the owner to pay for it. If there is fresh cabinetry which smells, sealing particle board surfaces and edges with two coats of special sealer will help.

What sort of particles are likely to make up the dust entering a street level or second-floor apartment?

Outdoor dust is largely made up of mineral and organic particles from soil and from plant materials such as pollens. There are also particles from thousands of other natural and human sources, including agriculture, industry, combustion and vehicles. Vehicle dust contains hazardous particles from brake linings and soot from poorly tuned engines, especially diesels.

In dry conditions dust travels readily with the slightest air current, and will enter your home or apartment. Allergenic dusts are a particular problem for those who suffer from hay fever or other sensitivities to plant materials, but many vehicle and industrial dusts are a concern for everyone. Street level and second-floor apartments are particularly vulnerable to dust problems from the street; above the second floor conditions usually improve dramatically. If you are on a lower floor and have a choice, ventilate with windows which face a rear yard, side yard or courtyard. In many cases it may be helpful to use a portable, high-efficiency air filter to clean both incoming air and recirculated air. It should contain both fine particle filters and odor removal filters. Apartments will also adsorb some odors from outside which have entered when the windows are open. These may take several hours or days of airing out, or air cleaning with a carbon filter to remove.

I am considering installing an electronic air filter in my furnace because I've heard that the conventional filters aren't very good. Will it help reduce dust levels?

Conventional furnace filters are not very effective for trapping small dust particles and are often poorly maintained. Curiously, a clogged filter is actually very good for trapping dust, but the fan just cannot force enough air through it to make it work effectively.

Electronic filters will trap much more of the fine dust than your conventional filter can without restricting airflow, but they will require regular maintenance. There is also a small hazard from ozone which is produced by these filters. It is a potent respiratory irritant. Newer filters produce less than older designs, but they still produce a bit of ozone. The collector plates must be removed and cleaned regularly to keep them working effectively and to reduce the ozone hazard. Electronic filters may also become noisy during use. High-voltage discharge sometimes makes them crackle and pop.

A simple and less costly way to improve air filtration with a furnace is to use a better performance filter in place of the basic furnace filters. These are available from air filtration equipment suppliers. Medium-efficiency filters, for example, are not electrical, but are simply better quality filters made of folded paper or fabric. These are rated from about 15% to 60% efficient by the Atmospheric Dust Spot Method. Be sure that any filter purchased is rated for use as a replacement in furnaces and remember to replace it as recommended. If you have an older furnace, you must verify that the fan is capable of handling the extra filter. If not, the fan may need to be replaced. Most pleated filters will last up to one year. If there is someone with environmental sensitivity disorder in your home, you may have to select a filter that is acceptable to the sensitive person. This will require some trial and error, as adhesives, filter fabric materials and treatments are varied, as are individual sensitivities.

What can I do about water pollution?

Depending on the source of water and the piping system, there can be many contaminants in your household water. If water comes from a local system, such as a well, spring, river, or lake, it can be contaminated by bacteria from surface runoff or sewage, parasites from animals, or it may contain dangerous chemicals from industrial waste, agriculture, automobiles or landfills. Some of these will be volatile and may have an odor. It is not only drinking water that is important. People absorb over 50% of the total dose of volatile water contaminants through the lungs and skin while showering because the shower head vaporizes the volatile contents. Chlorine compounds from chlorinated water and industrial solvents are absorbed this way.

For local water systems, a water test should be done to determine treatment needs. Also, a sterilizer (ultraviolet or ozone) should be used with any filter system for local water (especially surface sources), due to the potential for bacteria and parasites. A water quality expert or your local health department can help with deciding treatment needs.

If water comes from a municipal system, it is unlikely to contain dangerous bacteria, and if it contains industrial chemicals, they are likely to be at very low levels. It may, however, contain trace metals and sediments and it is almost certain to be chlorinated. Chlorine prevents bacterial contamination, but produces objectionable taste and odor. It combines chemically with organic material in water to form compounds such as chloroform and chloramine, which are health hazards. Acid water accelerates the breakdown of metal pipes and the solder used to join them, which may contain lead.

Water from a municipal system is tested regularly and a current water analysis report may be requested from the water district office. Have an expert look at it to determine what type of treatment is appropriate.

Water treatment can remove nearly all contaminants, but the right methods must be used. Fine particle filters and activated carbon are common devices for removing sediment and odors. Reverse osmosis is often used as well for minerals and organic compounds. There are special filters for removing dissolved heavy metals, and systems for removing iron and sulfur compounds. But buyer beware; there are a lot of false product claims and unscrupulous sales methods in the water treatment market.

Three other rules to remember: run the tap for a half minute to clear dissolved metals from pipes before taking drinking or cooking water if the water hasn't been used for several hours; avoid drinking or cooking with water from the hot tap; and if the water is hard, soften only the supply to the hot water heater.

Does a photocopier produce air pollution?

Yes it does. So does a laser printer or laser fax. These all produce ozone, an irritating gas generated by the high-voltage electrical fields inside the machines. Ozone is one of the components in smog which causes burning eyes and throat, and lung irritation. It may cause an asthma attack in some people. Photocopiers also produce fine dust and chemical vapors from the toner and heated fuser drum. They should always be used with ventilation, particularly in an enclosed space, or where two or more devices are placed together. An opening window may be adequate for a small office in mild weather, but an exhaust fan such as the type used for kitchens is best, particularly with several machines.

Are polyurethanes and lacquers safe?

The conventional urethane varnishes and colored plastic finishes use solvents which are volatile, but fairly stable once they have fully cured. This may take several weeks, depending on temperature and ventilation. Sensitive people may be bothered by them even a year later. Solvent-type lacquers (e.g. nitrocellulose) use a very volatile and intoxicating solvent, but they cure more quickly. Both types should be used with care, with adequate ventilation, and should be applied in a shop and cured before delivery if possible. If they must be used in place, the painter should use a respirator with special carbon adsorption filters and no one else should be in the area. Other special industrial finishes, such as melamines, epoxies and acrylic lacquers, should only be handled by fully qualified painters in a fully equipped paint shop.

In the past 10 years, whole new families of water-dispersed urethanes and lacquers have been developed which perform, handle and wear nearly as well as their solvent-based predecessors for some uses. These also contain solvents, but they are a safer type and less is used in the formulations. The two-part urethanes, called "cross linked," are very durable and will last at least as well as the old solvent type urethane, yet are safer to handle. Chemically sensitive people should carefully self-test any finish before deciding to use it. A fresh sample of the material should be applied to a clean piece of metal or glass, and then cured as recommended by the manufacturer. The individual should then bring it close, cautiously allowing a careful sniff. If it seems acceptable, it should be kept nearby for several days. A sample can also be put in a clean glass jar and sealed for several hours to discover if any odor accumulates.

Is plywood safe?

Exterior plywood produces only a small fraction of the formaldehyde generated by interior boards such as particle board and decorative plywood, though it does contain glues which have emissions. These glues are phenolic types, and may have a slight odor when fresh or when heated.

Exterior plywood is generally safe for interior use and is a good substitute for particle board in items such as cabinet frames and flooring underlays. A few people, however, may react to the tree resins (plant terpenes) released from the fir, pine and spruce softwoods often used for the plywood veneer. These people may tolerate small amounts of sealed plywood, or they may only be comfortable with solid hardwoods or hardwood plywood made with exterior glue.

Water board or strand board is often made with hardwoods which contain less terpenes, but they have a much higher glue content and tend to have a strong phenolic odor.

What can be done about mildew odors coming from a basement which has flooded?

Mildew is a fungus which grows in moist conditions. It can survive on a wide range of building materials and fabrics. Basements with raised wood floors on damp concrete often have severe fungus and dry rot problems which can affect the whole house through upward air movement. Any fungus growth is a health concern because some types are responsible for severe allergic reactions and even chronic diseases. Most fungi and their spores (seedlike particles) are irritating and allergenic. They also produce many gases which are irritants. Everyone should avoid massive exposure.

The first thing to do is to solve the drainage problem and dry the basement thoroughly, using heat and ventilation. Discard any carpet, fabric, wallboard or insulation that has become saturated, and clear out the space entirely. If the basement contains rotted wood it should be removed. A dilute solution of chlorine bleach (1/4 cup to a gallon of water, or 60 ml to 4 liters) is very effective for treating the flooded areas, but should be used with lots of ventilation and should be rinsed off. Hydrogen peroxide will help remove fungus stains if bleach is not acceptable to the occupants. After removing the stains, a solution of 1/2 cup of borax dissolved in a gallon of hot water (120 ml in 4 liters) is also effective for reducing the odor, and will retard future fungus growth if not entirely rinsed away. Once again, use ventilation and heat to dry the basement after treatment.

The basement should be isolated from the house as much as possible while cleanup is underway by taping the inside basement door closed and sealing off any heat vents or air returns in the basement which lead to a central heating system.

A strong ozone generator, available from fire and flood damage repair companies, can also be used in a sealed, unoccupied room for several hours to reduce residual odors and spores. Ozone is a very effective sterilizer and odor remover. After ozone treatment the room should be aired well for at least 12 hours to remove residual odors.

Is it a good idea to use an aerosol air freshener and disinfectant?

Air fresheners contain strong perfumes which are intended to create an impression of freshness, but which actually mask problem odors which should be recognized and dealt with. For example, soiled carpets, fungus problems or odors from smoking are not improved by air fresheners, they are just hidden. Furthermore, some aerosols contain chemicals, such as phenols and citrus and pine resins, which are more irritating to some people than the odor was in the first place.

There is little medical evidence to suggest that using aerosol disinfectants containing germicide in rooms reduces the incidence of illness. There may be a role for them where very infectious diseases are present, but in most situations they are ineffective. In fact, it is well known that continued use of disinfectants encourages the development of bacteria which can resist disinfectants.

Can underground water streams flowing under a house affect people's health?

Maybe. This concern is based on folk wisdom about "geomantic" or subtle forces flowing within the earth that can affect our health and well-being. The geomantic traditions go back for thousands of years in many cultures. They include the mystical practices of the ancient people of Britain, and the use of Feng Shui (wind and water energies) in Asia. These traditions have been brought forward today by a few people who practice dowsing and many forms of mystical healing, astrology and so on.

This area is clearly one where personal belief and philosophy is very important, as the concept of subtle energies is rejected outright by most people who claim to be rational. Curiously, however, some of the most advanced physics today is suggesting links between the observed world and much larger patterns and forces which transcend rational understanding. It is very likely that there are many forces at work around us which are not measurable, but which affect us nonetheless. It is also probably always a good idea to pay attention to folk wisdom. It is an important connection with the past, that often turns out to be more durable than current trends in science.

Can combustion gases enter a home from a water heater or furnace?

This is a common problem, especially in weather-sealed houses with older fuel-burning equipment. Any fuel-burning device requires a reliable chimney draft in order to discharge all of the gases resulting from combustion. Conventional chimneys take warm air from the home to maintain the draft. The burner also needs a source of outside air to supply oxygen for the flames. If the chimney is a conventional one of sheet metal or masonry, and it is sound and not blocked by any obstruction, and the furnace or water heater is properly installed, then the most important steps to prevent leakage are reliable sources of chimney draft and combustion air.

A fireplace is particularly prone to this problem, and can be reversed by a gust of wind or opening a door suddenly. This is especially true when the fire has nearly died out.

In houses which have been thoroughly draft sealed, all chimneys can be sluggish or even reverse when a powerful exhaust fan is turned on in the kitchen. This reversal also typically happens for at least a few seconds after the fuel ignites when the chimney is cold. One way to minimize this problem is to install a reasonably tight furnace room around the unit and provide a duct bringing outside air into the room. In very cold climates the air may have to be preheated in winter.

If the house is very airtight and has combustion appliances, the safest solution is to use the newer "sealed combustion" type burners. These units have an airtight chamber around the flame which is directly connected to a combustion air duct and a vent. This design minimizes the risk of combustion gas leakage due to chimney reversal. Though these cost more, they are also more efficient, and will eventually pay back their higher initial cost in fuel savings.

The draft of a conventional furnace or water heater can be checked by holding a smoldering taper made from rolled paper near the draft opening in the chimney pipe. The draft opening is a gap or special fitting in the vent pipe just above the appliance which allows room air to flow up the chimney to maintain the draft. The smoke should flow readily into the chimney and not be discharged back into the room, especially just after the burner starts. This should be tried again with the kitchen and bathroom exhaust fans operating. Smoke pencils, available from safety supply companies, are a better way to do this test, but they are also expensive and slightly hazardous. Hiring an air pollution testing company is the best option for many people.

Can a forced-air system be used for ventilation?

Yes, forced-air systems are very well suited to distribute ventilation because they have ducts to most rooms in the house. Forced-air systems are usually set up this way today, and older systems can be modified to ventilate. Ventilation is the removal of stale air from the house, usually from bathrooms, kitchens, laundries and basements, and its replacement by outdoor air. The furnace cannot effectively remove the exhaust from the house, but it can provide the outdoor air.

Every furnace should have a duct introducing outdoor air into the return plenum just before the filter. The outdoor air can be passed through an energy recovery ventilator and filtered first if so desired. This is not the same as providing combustion air for the furnace, though under some codes the combustion air is brought in the same way. This outdoor air supply should be sufficient to replace the air being exhausted elsewhere in the home by exhaust fans and natural convection, above and beyond the combustion air used by the burner. A qualified heating contractor should set up these supplies to ensure that they are safe and code approved.

What are the most immediate symptoms of environmentally induced illness?

Illnesses related to exposures in the environment often produce allergic or flu-like symptoms. Difficulty in breathing, congestion, sneezing, burning eyes and nose, itchy skin, sweating and skin rash are common signs. Headaches, drowsiness, dizziness, depression, nausea, muscle weakness, blurred vision and ringing ears also sometimes occur. In rare cases people may feel panic and even lose consciousness. The symptoms are connected to an exposure of some kind, and relief is found by removing the cause, though this may not happen immediately. The symptoms are *not* accompanied by a fever, which distinguishes environmental illness from a flu or other infection.

People who are said to be environmentally ill are a special group who are very reactive to many environmental conditions, often including tiny amounts of air pollution, common foods, lighting conditions, noise and so on. A person who is tired, depressed, weak, emotionally stressed and may be eating inappropriate foods is more susceptible to environmental illness. A person who has suffered a very traumatic illness or shock may also be a candidate. A person who has suffered acute or chronic exposure to toxic chemicals or potent drugs can also develop environmental illness. Many who have developed this condition have a history of exposure to hazardous chemicals in laboratories or hospitals, industry or agriculture.

259

A specialist physician should be consulted in all cases where these symptoms occur. If it seems that environmental causes are likely, a physician may suggest changes to environment, diet and habits, and may use tests, questionnaires and other methods to determine specific causes.

Can an office or apartment above a parking garage be affected by auto exhaust?

Auto exhaust and other air pollution from any source can move through buildings by routes that are not always immediately apparent. Many underground parking areas have exhaust fans which discharge at ground level near doors and windows, or near building air intakes. Some building air intakes are located above loading areas where trucks regularly stand idling for long periods. In extreme cases, carbon monoxide poisoning causing dizziness, depression, nausea and slowed reflexes will occur in the building.

In the case of an apartment, if there is no obvious outdoor path for air to move from the garage into the apartment, there is probably an indoor path such as a stairwell, corridor, elevator shaft or ventilation shaft. These will act like chimneys under certain conditions, drawing polluted air upward from the source. There are also numerous possible cracks and holes around pipes or wiring which can draw polluted air inward. These holes may be concealed in a wall or under a cabinet. In all buildings, openings between garages and occupied spaces are supposed to be sealed for fire safety.

Indoor pollution entry paths can be blocked with sealants or sheet metal if they can be found. If the pollutant is flowing up stairwells or elevators, fans can be installed to reverse the upward flow. Outdoor paths can be more difficult to stop, because apartments usually rely on open windows for ventilation.

Can gases seep into houses that have been built on landfills?

Yes, there are many paths through drains and foundation cracks which allow soil gases to enter. Gas entry is increased by heating and exhaust fans. If the landfill contains organic waste, such as municipal garbage and garden waste, it is likely to produce methane gas and possibly hydrogen sulfide. Methane is odorless, and explosive in high concentrations. It is the main constituent of the natural gas which is piped into homes, but natural gas has had an odorant added to it for safety. Methane is an asphyxiant which impairs normal breathing, and will cause drowsiness and headaches if allowed to build up indoors. Hydrogen sulfide smells very strongly of rotten eggs and is very toxic.

Gases from soils can be extracted by ventilation. It is best to ventilate the soil outside the foundation using perforated pipes buried in gravel. After this step, the basement can also be ventilated to dilute any gases which manage to enter. Often a fan is used to force air from an upper floor into the basement to maintain a slight positive pressure between the basement and the surrounding soil.

A more serious problem in homes built on landfill sites is the possibility that the site contains toxic wastes. Toxic waste seepage in soil and groundwater has been known to seriously contaminate homes with carcinogenic substances and other hazards. Common examples are waste oils, paints and solvents, pesticides and dry-cleaning fluids. These pollutants may also eventually enter groundwater and contaminate drinking water supplies.

The history of a site is a key piece of knowledge when considering a location. If there is a history of industrial dumping it is essential to know, because it can be very difficult to find a remedy for this problem once a building has been built. In most areas, the vendor of a property is required to disclose all knowledge of previous uses which may be hazardous.

Is natural gas safe?

Natural gas is a mixture of gases occurring naturally in underground petroleum formations. It consists mainly of methane, with small amounts of butane, propane and ethane gases, all of which are explosive and have little or no odor. It usually has traces of undesirable impurities also, such as hydrogen sulfide. Natural gas uses an odorizer additive, made from methyl and butyl mercaptans (also called methanethiol), that makes leaks noticeable.

In high concentrations, natural gas is an asphyxiant which interferes with normal breathing. Exposure to gas leaks usually causes nausea and headaches which clear up shortly after leaving the contaminated area. However, to some people who are environmentally sensitive, the slightest amount of gas can cause severe reactions ranging from dizziness to migraines and loss of muscle control. This can occur even in a kitchen where a gas burner is in use without proper exhaust, or where an appliance has a slight gas leak.

It is likely that the odorizer additive is at least partly responsible for these reactions, because natural gas itself is not highly toxic. Methyl mercaptan is listed as a dangerous substance, and even small exposures should be avoided.

The major health risk from the use of natural gas, other than fire or explosion, is the entry of combustion gases into the home from unvented stoves and heaters, and from malfunctioning chimneys. When gas burns it produces a wide range of toxic products, including carbon monoxide and nitrogen oxides. Carbon monoxide is a well-known asphyxiant which is particularly dangerous because it has no odor. It reduces the blood's ability to absorb oxygen, causing dizziness, headache, nausea, weakness, blurred vision, and loss of judgment and reflexes. Nitrogen oxides are respiratory irritants which cause burning nose and eyes, as well as coughing and choking sensations. Chronic exposure to nitrogen oxides causes breathing disorders and can also suppress the white blood cells, causing some loss of immunity to disease.

Every kitchen should have an efficient exhaust unit, and it should be used regularly, especially if a gas range is used. Chimneys should be checked by a qualified heating specialist, and unvented combustion of any kind should be avoided indoors.

How long does particle board outgas formaldehyde?

Indoor particle board used as flooring or carpet underlay and in cabinet and furniture frames is the major source of formaldehyde in most homes. Formaldehyde comes from the glue used in construction. It has a sharp, pungent odor and is very irritating, especially to those with respiratory difficulties. Minimizing sources such as particle board is the best way to reduce formaldehyde levels in homes. Where this is not practical, improving ventilation, sealing or neutralizing the source, or cleaning the air with an adsorbent filter may be helpful, but these are secondary strategies, not intended as a complete substitute for removing the source.

The rate of formaldehyde release from particle board diminishes with time. Within a few months it typically drops to half or less of what it was on the day of manufacture. After one or two years it is a small fraction of what it was when new. Formaldehyde release is accelerated by excess humidity and heat. There is a wide variation in the emission strength of various products due to differences in glue chemistry and quality control used by different manufacturers. This makes it difficult to know which are the safest, and to determine when the outgassing will be finished.

Manufacturers have reduced the formaldehyde emission rate from particle board over the past few years by better quality control, and products are now available bearing an HUD, label which indicates lower emissions. Boards meeting the more stringent European E1 label are even better. Better yet, there are boards made with alternative glues containing no formaldehyde at all.

Formaldehyde air testing is quite simple and inexpensive. Samplers can be ordered and returned for analysis, or an air quality consultant can do it. It is not wise to proceed with expensive renovations or replacement of furniture or cabinets without this information. Sealing particle board with two coats of lacquer or special formaldehyde sealer is moderately effective in reducing formaldehyde emissions. Sealing the entire surface of the board with a vapor-proof material such as plastic laminate or metal foil is very effective, but all edges and holes must be covered carefully.

Does light color affect health?

Yes it does, though it is more accurate to say that it primarily affects well-being. Light is necessary to activate some vitamins (to absorb calcium, for example) and to stimulate the brain signals which regulate mood. Most people get enough by short periods in full daylight, but some people need extra stimulation to prevent Seasonal Affective Disorder or, SAD, a depressed state in winter. This disorder is more common in northerly coastal regions with cloudy weather and short winter days. About 20 minutes spent daily under a very bright lamp seems to help these people when no sunlight or bright daylight is available.

There are also claims that full spectrum lamps, and lamps containing ultraviolet light are better for health. These lamps are much closer to daylight than the light from a common incandescent lamp or cool white fluorescent lamp. Of course the color spectrum of lighting affects the way skin and hair appears, and so obviously affects accurate perception and ambiance. It probably also affects mood in subtle ways, but there is little evidence that color balance and ultraviolet components are directly beneficial to health. Most people get enough bright light from daily activity, indoors and out. Lighting color, brightness and ambiance are most important in hospitals, schools and for office work where people spend long periods inside.

Daylight and access to an outdoors view is perhaps an even more important human need than is color balanced lighting. It helps to provide orientation, a natural sense of time, and appreciation of changes in weather and outdoor activity.

Can ozone or negative ions clean the air and improve health?

Ozone is a very potent and irritating gas which is produced by an electrical discharge such as lightning. It is simply a recombination of the oxygen molecules which exist in air. It lasts for only a few minutes at most, and is capable of reacting with volatile gases which cause odors and with microorganisms such as fungus spores and bacteria. The result is that the odors are reduced dramatically and many of the spores and bacteria are sterilized so that they are no longer active. Ozone is sometimes applied at high levels in a sealed, unoccupied room using an electric ozone generator for neutralizing smoke odors, particularly from fire damage. It also works for odors from mildew damage and from some materials, such as fresh paint, plastic or new carpet, which emit volatile gases.

An ozone generator is also sometimes offered as a room air cleaner for occupied rooms, or as a device to fit into furnace ducts to "improve air quality." Adding ozone to occupied rooms is probably not a good idea in any case. One problem with ozone is that it can induce asthma attacks in sensitive people. Another problem is that it paralyzes the ability to smell. It is therefore difficult to know if an elevated ozone level in an occupied room is simply masking an odor rather than neutralizing it. It may not be possible for sensitive people to tolerate high enough ozone exposures to actually have much effect on odors and microorganisms. It is probably best to avoid ozone exposures in occupied buildings altogether.

An ion generator alters the balance of negatively and positively charged ions which occur naturally in air. It is known that there is typically a deficit of negative ions indoors, and that some people experience an elevated mood or sense of alertness, breathing comfort and well-being if the negative ion level is increased. However, the effect is not well understood, and it doesn't seem to work for everyone. It is probably safe to use ion generators in occupied rooms, because no ill effects are known.

Why does a building often smell contaminated near the entry?

Sometimes there really is an air quality problem which is localized near the entry, such as mildewed clothing or floor coverings damaged by moisture and soil, or contaminated air entering from outside. But more often there really isn't much difference between the entrance and other rooms. When we step into a building from outside, the differences in odors between outdoors and indoors is immediately apparent, but the ability to distinguish only lasts about 15 to 30 seconds. After that, the senses have become adapted to the new conditions and we can no longer compare with outdoors. To check this observation, try another room which has an opening window or balcony. Stand for a few minutes with your head outside and breathe deeply, then step inside and compare.

Glossary

Acetate: A chemical structure, usually referring to cellulose acetate fiber or film, or vinyl acetate used in adhesives.

Acetone: A very volatile and toxic solvent used in lacquers, inks and adhesives, and for cleaning painting equipment.

Acrylic impregnated flooring: Prefinished sheet flooring system that has had liquid acrylic forced under pressure into its porous structure. The acrylic hardens, forming an extremely abrasion-resistant finish, throughout the full thickness. Dyes and fire retardants may be added.

Acrylic polymers: A family of plastic materials used for rigid plastic sheets (Plexiglas), liquid coatings (floor wax and sealers), paints and many other products. Acrylics are made from acrylic acids, methacrylate, or acrylonitrile, all derived from petroleum. Acrylics are relatively low in toxicity, but the solvents associated with acrylic paints may not be.

Admixtures or additives (concrete): Minor ingredients, mixed with concrete to impart particular properties, such as color, decreased drying time or improved workability.

Air barriers: An air barrier is a means of restricting the movement of air into insulated cavities. It may also incorporate a vapor barrier. Polyethylene sheet, joined with tape or caulking, is the most common type. Airtight drywall is another type.

Airtight drywall: A system of joining interior panels of gypsum, plywood or other rigid materials using gaskets and caulking, to restrict air movement into insulated cavities. This method provides a highly durable and reliable air barrier and vapor barrier, far superior to polyethylene sheet methods.

Aliphatic hydrocarbons: A large family of chemicals based on hydrogen and carbon atoms connected in straight or branched chains. Aliphatics include many paraffins and oils, petroleum derivatives, and bases for many plastics. *See also* Aromatic hydrocarbons.

Allergen: Any substance capable of producing an allergic response, especially in sensitive persons. Some common allergens are proteins contained in pollens, grains, fungi, nuts and seeds.

Ammonia: A very irritating and potentially toxic gas (NH3), which is the basis of a large number of industrial chemicals and fertilizers. Easily dissolved in water, ammonia is a common component of latex paints and household cleaners. Ammonia is also produced naturally by bacterial action on urea.

Ammonia fumigation: A process using ammonia gas to neutralize formaldehyde emissions from such materials as particle board and adhesives. *See also* Hexamethylenetetramine.

Ammonium sulfide: Usually refers to ammonium bisulfide, a hazardous and irritating chemical used in textile dyeing and treatment.

Antibacterial: See Bactericide.

Aromatic hydrocarbons: A large family of chemicals based on hydrogen and carbon atoms which form ring-shaped molecules. Many aromatics evaporate readily and have strong odors (e.g. toluene and xylene). Many are toxic or carcinogenic (e.g. benzene).

Asbestos: A family of mineral fibers found in certain types of rock formations. Asbestos is very fireproof and resistant to chemical attack. It has been used in insulation, plaster, floor tiles and concrete pipe. The fibers are very hazardous if inhaled or swallowed, and cause lung cancer, chest cancer, asbestosis (a lung disease), and other forms of cancer. Of the several types of asbestos, crocidolite is the most dangerous, and chrysotile the least. Asbestos use has been severely restricted in building materials and consumer products since the early 1970s.

Asphalt-treated paper: A facing on some batt insulation that provides a barrier to moisture, consisting of paper coated with asphalt (derived from petroleum by-products).

Backdrafting (back venting or flue gas spillage): A conventional chimney serving a furnace, heater or fireplace depends on the buoyancy of warm combustion gases to carry them outside. This is a weak force, and can easily be overcome by a strong exhaust fan in a house, or by wind conditions, particularly when the chimney is cold. When this occurs, these hazardous gases enter the home.

Backed vinyls or laminated vinyls: Consist of a surface wear layer of vinyl and a backing layer, usually of fabric, paper or plastic foam.

Bactericide: Any agent which will destroy bacteria. Bactericides are commonly added to water-based paints, waxes and other consumer products to prevent spoilage. They are toxic materials which are usually only safe in very low concentrations. *See also* Biocide; Fungicide.

Barrier cloth: A special synthetic or cotton fabric that does not allow dust to penetrate. It has a very high thread count (300 per inch), and is tightly woven.

Batt or blanket insulation: Glass or mineral wool which may be faced with paper, aluminum, or another vapor barrier. For use in building cavities.

Bentonite: An aluminum silicate clay capable of great expansion when wet. Used in ceramics, paper coatings, waterproofing, foods and cosmetics. Low toxicity.

Benzene: A carbon and hydrogen compound with a ring-shaped molecule. One of the most common building blocks for synthetic chemicals. Generally derived from petroleum, benzene is highly toxic and carcinogenic. *See also* Aromatic hydrocarbon.

Binder: Any material used to hold another together or make it more adhesive. Binders are usually synthetic polymers and are commonly used in coatings to form a film when dry.

Biocide or biostat: An additive which will prevent growth of bacteria or fungi. Biocides are used in paints, floor coverings and sometimes in fabrics. They are toxic materials which are usually only safe in very low concentrations.

Biodegradable: A material which can be decomposed when discarded by the normal action of bacteria and fungi. Typical examples are paper and wood products, natural fibers and starches.

Boric acid, boron salt: Naturally occurring compounds containing boron. Commonly used in household cleaners and as fungicides in consumer products. Boron-based fungicides are much safer than their mercury-based or biphenyl counterparts.

Breathability: The ability of a finish to allow moisture to escape from behind the film without causing blistering or peeling.

Building-related illness: See Sick building syndrome

Cadmium: A soft, easily molded heavy metal, used in pigments and heat stabilizers in the vinyl-making process. It is quite toxic and causes permanent kidney and liver damage. Cadmium accumulates in the environment.

Calcination: The heating of minerals to concentrate them, and remove moisture or volatile compounds, e.g. gypsum is calcined to make plaster of Paris.

Calcium carbonate: The mineral base of limestone, marble, seashells and chalk. Calcium carbonate is heated to form lime (calcium oxide). Very low toxicity.

Carcinogen: Any naturally occurring or synthetic substance known to increase the risk of cancer.

Carnauba: A wax derived from the Brazilian wax palm leaf. Used in paste waxes, furniture polish, plastics and food glazes. Very low toxicity.

Casein (calcium caseinate, sodium caseinate): The protein base of milk. Casein is used as a base and binder in natural paints and adhesives. It is a very low toxicity material, but is allergenic to people with milk sensitivities.

Cellulose: The natural carbohydrate base for plant fibers, it is the most abundant organic material in the world. Used to make paper and textiles.

Cembra pine: Also known as Swiss pine, its resin has inherent pesticide properties.

Cementitious: Any material based on cement or cement-like products, i.e. inorganic, noncombustible, and hard-setting.

Chemically stable materials: Those which will not readily break down or release (potentially toxic) chemicals with the influence of other chemicals, age, heat or light.

Chemical sensitivity: A loosely defined condition experienced by some people who are affected by very small concentrations of chemicals in air, water and food, which would not have apparent effects on most people. Symptoms may be similar to minor allergies, though they may also include moderate to severe pains, muscle weakness, dizziness, confusion and even seizures.

Chemical sensitization: The process of becoming sensitive to chemicals through excessive exposure, e.g. to fungi, wood dusts or formaldehyde.

Chipboard or particle board: A building panel consisting of wood chips and fibers pressed together, using a synthetic resin as a binding agent.

Chlorinated compounds: A large family of synthetic chemicals which are formed by combining chlorine with hydrocarbons. Many, such as DDT, are environmental toxins and very persistent. Some, such as dry cleaning solvents (e.g. perchloroethylene), present serious disposal problems. Many are toxic or carcinogenic, and will accumulate in fat tissues, liver and kidneys. *See also* Chlorofluorocarbons.

Chlorofluorocarbons (CFCs): Synthetic chemicals manufactured from hydrocarbons and chlorine, fluorine or bromine. Commonly used as refrigerants and solvents, all have some potential to destroy ozone in the upper atmosphere when released. Most are very chemically stable, and some are toxic. Most are being phased out by international ozone treaty.

Coalescing solvent: A solvent that causes two or more substances to combine, e.g. a solvent which causes a paint to harden.

Convection: Convection is the movement of a liquid or a gas such as air due to the changes in density at different temperatures. For example, when air is heated it becomes less dense and is then pushed up by cold air around it. An example of natural convection is warm air rising in a room and collecting near the ceiling.

Copolymer: See Polymer.

Curing: The process and time period for a finish to achieve its final state of hardness, color, etc. A chemical reaction is usually involved.

Damp-proofing: A treatment, such as a sealer or asphalt coating, that inhibits the transfer of moisture in foundations.

Dimethyl ether: An ether made from wood alcohol used as a solvent and propellent in spray cans. Moderate toxicity but very flammable.

Dispersion: A mixture in which solids are suspended in a liquid, e.g. paint, usually in small globules.

Dolomitic: Limestone or chalk materials made up from carbonate rocks. Very low toxicity. *See also* Calcium carbonate.

Dry adhesives: Factory-applied adhesives that adhere with pressure and remain flexible. Usually low toxicity.

Drying oil: An oil, such as linseed or synthetic oil, which contains additives causing it to harden when exposed to air. Usually used in paints.

Efflorescence: The formation of white crystals on the surface of concrete, mortar, tile or brick, caused by leaching of mineral salts. It is not hazardous.

Elastomer: A rubberlike material which will remain flexible, used to fill cracks, join other materials which may move over time, and where resilience is important. Caulkings are elastomers, as are soft rubber and plastics. *See also* Polymer.

Emissions: Releases of gases from any process or material. Liquid emissions are commonly referred to as effluents.

Emulsion: See Dispersion

Epichlorohydrin: A very toxic and carcinogenic substance used in manufacturing epoxies, some synthetic rubbers, and other adhesives.

Epoxy: A class of synthetic resins used for high-performance adhesives, paints, and protective coatings. Epoxy adhesives and paints are two-part materials mixed immediately before use. The ingredients are hazardous and should be handled only by those with training.

Ethyl alcohol: Grain alcohol, sometimes used as a solvent in paints and waxes, and in dyeing processes. Ethyl alcohol is intoxicating when ingested, but the vapor is relatively harmless.

Ethylene glycol: An alcohol, often used as a solvent in water- and oil-based paints, lacquers and stains. Toxic when ingested or inhaled, ethylene glycol is also the main ingredient of automotive antifreeze.

Fan-coil: A furnace containing a fan and low-temperature heat exchange coil and filters, but no burner.

Feldspar: A natural, silica mineral used in glassmaking and ceramic glazes.

Ferric oxide: Oxide of iron (rust). Used for pigment in paints. Very low toxicity.

Fiberboards: Construction panels made from compressed fibers, including wood, paper, straw or other plant fibers. Three common types are:

- High density—highly compressed fiber, usually made with no added adhesive. May also be "tempered" to provide an even harder surface. Commonly used for furniture backs, interior doors, industrial flooring and pegboard. Low toxicity.
- Medium density (MDF)—moderately compressed fiber held together with glue. Commonly used for cabinet and furniture frames, carpet underlay and as a core for decorative laminate paneling. Toxicity depends on adhesive.
- Low density—slightly compressed fiber, usually with no added adhesive. Commonly used for insulating sheathing, acoustic panels and tack boards. Low toxicity.

Fiberglass resin: Uncured polyester resin used for fabricating glass fiber reinforced and cast plastic products. Irritating and toxic to handle.

Fiberization: The process of reducing a material, such as newspaper or cotton, into a loose fiber for insulation or upholstery filling.

Filler: A material of little or no plasticity which adds bulk to paints or plastics, or helps to promote drying and control shrinkage in clay bodies.

Fire retardant or flame retardant: A substance added to a flammable material to reduce its flammability. It is only possible for fire retardants to slow the spread of fire; they do not make flammable materials fireproof. Used in fabrics, carpets, bedding, upholstery and foamed plastics, some are irritating or hazardous, such as phosphates and chlorinated compounds.

Foamed-in-place: An insulating material containing cements or plastics which is installed wet using foaming equipment.

Formaldehyde: A pungent and irritating gas used in the manufacture of many adhesives and plastics, as a preservative, and in permanent press fabrics. Many people suffer health effects from formaldehyde at very low concentrations. Formaldehyde is now listed as a suspected carcinogen.

Formaldehyde scavengers: Agents added to wood products manufactured with formaldehyde-based glues to neutralize gases before they escape. Usually sulfite or ammonia compounds, scavengers are sometimes used to treat affected buildings directly by fumigation, or as a coating for air filters.

Fungi (molds, mildew, mushrooms): Plantlike organisms which do not require light for growth and survival because they do not produce chlorophyll. A few fungi are safe and edible, such as some species of mushrooms, while most produce very allergenic spores and odors.

Fungicide: Any substance added to inhibit the growth of fungus and consequent spoilage of a material. Paints, stucco, floor coverings, treated wood and outdoor fabrics are commonly treated with fungicides. Many are hazardous metal or chlorine compounds. Safer fungicides are usually boron or sulfate based. *See also* Biocide.

Glass fiber: Glass which has been extruded (stretched) while molten to make very fine fibers for insulation, and nonflammable fabrics or reinforced plastics. Glass fibers are irritating to the skin and dangerous if inhaled, though not as hazardous as asbestos.

Glycols: A family of alcohols used as solvents in many paints, coatings, etc. Some glycols are very safe while others are toxic. *See also* Ethylene glycol; Propylene glycol.

Grout: A cementitious material used to fill the joints between tiles. May contain acrylic or epoxy additives for greater durability.

Heat recovery ventilator (energy recovery ventilator or heat exchanger): A ventilator which contains a means of extracting heat from one air stream and transferring it to another.

Heavy metals: The series of metals including mercury, lead, cadmium, thallium, cobalt, nickel and aluminum. Most are very toxic and persistent in the environment. Mercury and lead accumulate in tissue and cause nervous system damage, cobalt and thallium are extremely toxic, cadmium is toxic to the kidneys and liver, aluminum is associated with Alzheimer's disease, and nickel is carcinogenic.

Hexamethylenetetramine (methenamine, aminoform or hexamine): A stable, crystalline substance formed by the action of ammonia on formaldehyde. It is the residue of formaldehyde neutralization which remains in wood products and buildings fumigated with ammonia. It is a skin irritant but is relatively low in toxicity.

Hexane (n-hexane): A solvent derived from petroleum, used in adhesives and paints. Hexane is moderately hazardous in low concentrations, causing symptoms of nerve toxicity, such as numbness, trembling or disorientation.

Hydrocarbons: A vast group of naturally occurring and synthetic compounds based on hydrogen and carbon atoms only. The primary source of the world's hydrocarbons is fossil fuels. Hydrocarbons are used as fuels and as feedstocks for most organic chemical synthesis. *See also* Aliphatic hydrocarbons; Aromatic hydrocarbons.

Hydrogenated chlorofluorocarbons (HCFCs or HFCs): Hydrogenated chlorofluorocarbons (or hydrogenated fluorocarbons) are substitute refrigerants and solvents which do not have as much potential to destroy atmospheric ozone if released as do CFCs. Most are less efficient as refrigerants than CFCs and some are quite toxic. *See also* Chlorofluorocarbons.

Hydrogen sulfide (H2S): A poisonous and odorous gas found in natural gas deposits, and produced by bacteria when decomposing waste without oxygen present. Gypsum building products present a disposal problem in wet climates because hydrogen sulfide is produced by bacteria when gypsum is buried.

Inorganic compound: Any compound which does not contain carbon atoms in its structure. Minerals, metals, ceramics and water are examples of inorganic compounds. Most tend to be very stable and persistent because they oxidize slowly or not at all. *See also* Organic compound.

Isocyanate: Similar to Isocyanurate, below.

Isocyanurate: A family of resins, usually called polyurethanes, which are used for insulating and upholstery foams, paints and varnishes. Because isocyanurates contain a cyanide group in their chemical structure, most will release deadly cyanide gas if exposed to a fire. At room temperature they are relatively nontoxic.

Isoparaffinic hydrocarbons: A type of highly purified petroleum solvent sold as "odorless paint thinner." Often used in solvent-based, low-toxicity paints, it is one of the safest solvents because the odorous portions which have been removed are also the most hazardous.

Joint compound: A wet filler material used to join materials of the same type, to create a uniform surface, e.g. gypsum filler.

Ketones: A chemical structure common to many solvents, such as acetone and methyl ethyl ketone.

Kiln dried: A method of drying wood in an oven after sawing that results in 10% or less moisture content. This makes the wood more dimensionally stable and better able to resist fungus in storage.

Lacquer: A glossy liquid finish for woods or metals, traditionally prepared from plant resins. Nitrocellulose lacquer, made from wood or cotton fiber treated with acid and dissolved in butyl acetate (lacquer thinner) is a more typical formulation today. Lacquer also refers to many types of hard, high-gloss industrial finishes, such as acrylic auto finishes.

Laminate: A thin layer of material (veneer) bonded to another surface. Wood and plastics are both commonly laminated.

Latex: A naturally occurring, sticky resin from rubber tree sap used for rubber products, carpet backings and paints. Latex is a broad term which also can apply to synthetic rubbers, usually styrene butadiene. *See also* Styrene butadiene rubber.

Lignin: A naturally occurring polymer in wood which keeps the fibers bound together. Most lignin is removed during papermaking and is burned as fuel. Pulped wood which has not had the lignin removed can be pressed into high-density fiberboard without adhesives, because the lignin will bind the fibers.

Linseed oil: Oil from the seed of the flax plant. Used in paints, varnishes, linoleum and synthetic resins. Nontoxic.

Loosefill insulation: Vermiculite, perlite, glass or mineral wool, shredded wood and paper. For use in building cavities and insulated ceilings.

Mastic: Refers to many synthetic caulkings and adhesives used for floors and tile laying. *See also* Elastomer.

Material Safety Data Sheet (MSDS): A legal requirement for all potentially hazardous products, the data sheet indicates the risks from using and disposing of the product and recommends safe practices. The sheet may also indicate the chemical contents of the product.

MDF: See Fiberboards

Melamine: A polymer used for plastics and paints made from formaldehyde, ammonia and urea. Similar to urea formaldehyde resin. Nontoxic if heat cured.

Methyl alcohol: Also called wood alcohol or methanol, it can be made by heating wood or peat under pressure, but is usually made from natural gas (methane). It is far more toxic than ethyl alcohol (grain alcohol) and is used in traditional shellacs, waxes and paints.

Methyl cellulose: A product of wood pulp used as a thickener, adhesive and food additive. Very low toxicity.

Methylene chloride: A solvent and paint remover. Very toxic and a known carcinogen.

Methyl ethyl ketone: A common solvent used in lacquers, paint removers and adhesives. Moderately toxic. Methyl ethyl ketone peroxide is a related compound, used as a hardener for fiberglass resin. It is toxic.

Mica: A naturally occurring silica mineral used as a filler in paints, gypsum fillers, and as electrical insulation. Low toxicity, but the dust is hazardous.

Micron: A unit of measurement, one thousandth of a millimeter.

Microorganism: Any microscopic living thing, such as a bacterium or fungus.

Mortar: A cement-based mixture used to lay stone or ceramic tiles, or for use as a grout for these materials.

Mothproofing: A treatment applied to fibers (usually wool) to resist damage by moths. Mothproofings are typically skin irritants and may cause adverse reactions on contact.

Mutagenic: A substance which is known to alter the genetic material (DNA) of cells, potentially causing changes in tissue growth leading to cancers.

Natural: A substance or material which is taken from nature as directly as possible with minimal intervention of processing or chemical synthesis.

Though not all natural materials are safe, their properties are well known through traditional uses.

Natural ventilation: Natural ventilation is air change provided by opening windows, or air leakage through the building envelope. Natural ventilation needs a driving force such as temperature differences between various parts of the house, or air pressure differences caused by wind.

Neoprene: Trade name for polychloroprene, a synthetic rubber used to manufacture caulking, rubber gaskets and waterproof membranes. Very odorous.

Nitrocellusose lacquer: See Lacquer

Nylon: Any of a family of polyamide resins used for textile fiber, rope and molded plastics. The most common type in carpet manufacture is Nylon 66, though Nylon 6 is also used.

Offgassing (or outgassing): The release of gases or vapors from solid materials. It is a form of evaporation, or a slow chemical change, which will produce indoor air pollution for prolonged periods after installation of a material.

Organically grown: Grown with minimal use of synthetic fertilizers or pesticides. Various state and industry definitions are used to determine which products can be sold as organically grown.

Organic compound: Any chemical compound based on the carbon atom. Organic compounds are the basis of all living things; they are also the foundation of modern polymer chemistry. There are several million known and their characteristics vary widely.

Organochlorine (organobromine, or organofluorine): Organic compounds formed with chlorine, bromine or fluorine in their structure. Organochlorines are usually either very toxic and persistent in nature (dioxins, PCBs, DDT) or very chemically stable (PVC, Teflon).

Oriented strand board (OSB): A manufactured wood product, mainly used in construction, composed of strands of wood laid in the same direction and glued together. This process produces a very high-strength product from low-grade waste material from the wood milling industry. Toxicity depends on adhesive.

Paraffin wax: A low-toxicity petroleum wax used in some finishes and for making candles. Approved as a food additive.

Parge: The application of stucco or mortar to a surface for protection.

Parquet: A small wooden tile made from interlocked strips of hardwood, and used as a floor covering. Parquet is usually glued down and varnished, or it may be prefinished.

Particulates: Particles of dust, mold, mildew, etc. small enough to become suspended in air. Very small particulates (less than .005 millimeter) can be inhaled deep into the lungs. Particulates containing plant or animal proteins are allergenic, while those containing mineral fiber (silica, asbestos) cause lung disease or cancer.

Parts per million: A unit of measurement for very small concentrations of gases or liquids. One part per million indicates a concentration of one million to one by volume.

Penetrating/impregnating sealer: A finish that will penetrate the porous structure of wood or tile, and protect not only the surface, but the entire upper layer of the material.

Perchloroethylene (PERC): A dry cleaning solvent and degreasing solvent. Hazardous to handle and dispose of. Vapor is toxic.

Perlite: A volcanic glass which is expanded and used as a plaster additive and fire-resistant insulation.

Petrochemicals: Any chemicals synthesized from petroleum. All are hydrocarbons. *See also* Hydrocarbons.

pH: An index of the acidity or alkalinity of a substance. A pH of 1 is highly acidic, 7 is neutral, and 13 is highly alkaline.

Phenol formaldehyde: An adhesive resin used for exterior plywood and other wood products. Dark brown in color and low in formaldehyde emissions.

Phenols (phenolic odor): A hydrocarbon with a ring structure, derived from oil or coal. Used to synthesize a large number of resins, glues and pharmaceuticals, and as a germicide. Very toxic.

Phenyl mercuric acetate: An organic compound of mercury previously used as a fungicide in paints, but now banned for most interior paints. A highly toxic material which does nerve damage.

Plasticizer: A chemical such as a phthalate added to a plastic or rubber to keep it soft and flexible, particularly common in vinyl upholstery and flexible floor coverings. The plasticizers offgas slowly.

Polyamide resin: The family of synthetic resins called nylons. *See also* Nylon.

Polyester: Any long chain polymers made from esters of alcohols. Fibers, solid and sheet plastics of many kinds are classified as polyester.

Polyethylene: A chemically simple, semitransparent plastic. Used widely as vapor barrier sheet over insulation, for packaging film, and containers. There are both high-density (HDPE) and low-density (LDPE) varieties. It is a low-toxicity material and produces low-risk vapors when it is burned.

Polyethylene terephthalate (PET): A polyester resin used to produce polyester fiber and sheet plastics, e.g. recyclable soft drink bottles.

Polymer or copolymer: Any of a large number of natural or synthetic, usually organic compounds composed of very large molecules chemically linked together in long chains. Cellulose and proteins are naturally occurring polymers. Plastics are synthetic polymers.

Polyolefin: A class of common, synthetic plastics including polyethylene and polypropylene. Polyolefin can be spun into fibers to produce a tough exterior weather barrier fabric for construction.

Polypropylene: A polyolefin with good flexibility used for carpet yarn, rope, artificial turf, packaging and primary carpet backing. It has a very smooth surface texture and tends to produce abrasive textiles.

Polystyrene: A plastic used in foamed building insulation or for tough, molded plastic products. Low toxicity, but contains toxic flame retardants.

Polyurethane: See Isocyanurate

Polyvinyl acetate (PVA): A plastic usually used in water-based emulsion glues, such as white glue, and in waxes and flooring adhesives. Relatively low toxicity.

Polyvinyl chloride (PVC): A chlorinated vinyl plastic which is very durable and chemically stable unless plasticized to keep it soft. The basis of most flexible flooring, plastic upholstery and plastic siding. Produced in a closed process using vinyl chloride, a very hazardous material. Vapors are hazardous when it is burned.

Portland cement: A kind of cement made by burning limestone and clay in a kiln. It is the base for most concrete, mortar and floor tile grouts.

Primer: First coat applied to a substrate, serving as a sealer and providing a good base for finishing coats.

Propylene glycol: An oily alcohol used in paints, waxes and sealers. Unlike ethylene glycol it is low toxicity, and approved as a food additive.

Radiant: Heat which is transferred between surfaces without contact or heating of air in between. Radiant heating in buildings requires a large surface heated to above body temperature.

Radon: A colorless, odorless, radioactive gas occurring naturally in soil and rock. Radon exposure increases risk of lung cancer. Most radon enters homes through basements and floor drains.

Recirculation: Recirculation is the movement of air inside the building without exchange with outdoor air. Recirculation is typically done to mix and distribute heated or cooled air, as well as to filter, humidify and dehumidify it. Recirculation is not a form of ventilation.

Relative humidity: Relative humidity (RH) is a measure of the moisture content of air compared to the maximum amount of moisture which the air could carry at that temperature. Relative humidity is expressed as a percentage, with 100 percent RH indicating air which is fully saturated with moisture. RH is an important factor in comfort and air quality. The healthiest range is between about 25% and 60%.

Resilient: Rubber, vinyl and linoleum floor coverings are called resilient because they are elastic.

Resin: A sticky substance that flows from certain plants and trees, especially pine and fir. It is used in paints and varnish. Artificial resins, used in the manufacture of plastics and synthetic finishes, are usually petroleum-based polymers.

Rigid insulation: Insulation materials, such as foamed plastic, wood, cork, glass or mineral fibers pressed into a standard-sized board for easy handling. Used as a surface insulation.

Rock wool or mineral wool: Insulating material spun from heated slag (waste), from metal smelting. Similar to glass fiber. The fiber is very irritating to the skin, and hazardous if inhaled.

R-value: Thermal insulating value, that is, the inverse of the rate of heat flow through a material. A high R-value indicates a low rate of heat transfer.

Sheathing: Rigid sheet material used to cover the framework of buildings or cabinets. Usually structural.

Shellac: Purified lac (a resin from a beetle), used for making varnishes and leather polishes. It is dissolved in methyl alcohol, and can also be thinned with safer ethyl alcohol. Low toxicity.

Sick building syndrome: A pattern of health complaints related to poor indoor air quality. Symptoms include eye, nose and throat irritation, nausea, fatigue, depression, headaches and skin irritations. The symptoms disappear when away from the affected building for hours or days.

Silicates: Compounds based on the element silicon, a very common component of sand and rock. Silicates are hazardous if inhaled but make very chemically stable building products.

Siliconate: Any of a large family of chemicals based on silica, e.g. silicic acid, sodium silicate, silicone.

Silicone: Organic compounds of silicon used for caulkings and flexible plastics, lubricating oils and sealers. A very low toxicity material.

Sizing: Sizing is a liquid surface treatment that seals the surface against absorption of adhesive and provides "tooth" for the wall covering. Sizing also refers to a temporary, formaldehyde-based fabric treatment which makes fabric stiffer and easier to work with. Fabric sizing is very irritating to some people.

Sodium fluorosilicate: A toxic compound used as a pesticide and preservative, and in dyeing processes. It is a popular mothproofing agent for wool.

Sodium silicate: Also called "water glass," a caustic liquid used for gluing cardboard, high-temperature cements, and sealing asbestos fibers. Also used in foamed insulation.

Styrene-butadiene rubber (SBR): A synthetic latex formed from petroleum and used for carpet backings and elastic fabrics. SBR has a characteristic pungent odor and releases several irritating gases.

Subfloor: The structural floor under a finished floor. Subfloors are usually made from plywood or diagonal boards.

Substrate: A material that provides the surface on which an adhesive is spread for any purpose, such as laminating or coating.

Surfactant: A surface active agent, useful for its cleaning, wetting or dispersing powers. Usually nontoxic.

Synthetic: Produced by chemical methods, i.e. not extracted from natural sources.

Terpenes: Organic, aromatic substances contained in the sap of softwoods. Terpenes can be highly irritating to sensitive people.

Terrazzo flooring: Marble or granite chips embedded in a binder that may be cementitious, noncementitious (epoxy, polyester or resin), or a combination of both. Can be used with divider strips of brass, zinc or plastic.

Thermoplastics: Plastic resins which can be molded when heated and retain their shape when cooled.

Thermosetting: Plastic resins which become hard and rigid after hot molding, and cannot be softened again with heat.

Thickset method: Mortar installation procedure used for uneven material, such as ungauged stone. The mortar bed is 3/4 in. to 1–1/4 in. thick (2 cm to 3 cm).

Thinset method: Installation procedure used for evenly gauged material, such as ceramic or granite tile. A mortar as thin as 3/32 in. (.24 cm) is used, often containing an acrylic adhesive.

Titanium dioxide: A white pigment used in paint, vitreous enamel, linoleum, rubber and plastics, printing ink and paper. It has low toxicity but high covering power, brilliance, reflectivity, and resistance to light and fumes. Production creates large quantities of toxic waste.

Toluene: An aromatic component of petroleum with a strong solvent odor. Moderately toxic and used as a solvent for adhesives and inks.

Toxic: Any substance which causes harm to living organisms. There is a wide range of toxicity, from very low to extremely toxic.

Traditional materials: Materials which have been used for several generations. Their properties and toxicity are known from experience.

Trichloroethane, 1,1,2 and 1,1,1: Potent solvents used in paints and inks, and as cleaning and degreasing fluids. 1,1,2 trichloroethane is sweet smelling and quite toxic. 1,1,1 trichloroethane, by contrast, is much less toxic.

Trichloroethylene: A solvent used in degreasing, dry cleaning, paints and adhesives. Moderately toxic, and classed as hazardous waste.

Tung oil: Oil obtained from the seed of the tung tree, widely used as a drying oil in paints and varnishes, and as a waterproofing agent.

Ultraviolet (UV): Short-wavelength, high-energy invisible light responsible for sunburn, skin cancer, and bleaching and deterioration of many materials.

Undercushion: A padding material laid prior to laying a carpet. Foamed plastic, rubber and felts are the most common types. All tend to capture dust and deteriorate with time.

Underlay: A sheet material, usually wood or wood fiber, laid under resilient flooring, carpet or tile to minimize irregularities in the subfloor or to add acoustic separation.

Urea formaldehyde: An inexpensive polymer used widely as glue for interior wood products. A source of toxic formaldehyde gas.

Urethane: See also Isocyanurate.

Vapor barrier: In addition to the moisture carried into building cavities by air movement, a small amount is also transferred by vapor diffusion. Because water vapor tends to move from a moist area to a dryer one, it can be forced through permeable materials such as wood and plaster. A vapor barrier is a material such as plastic film or impermeable paint which resists moisture movement in materials.

Veneer: A thin sheet of high-grade wood formed by cutting a thin strip from it. The veneer is applied to thicker wood or paper to make plywood and decorative wood-surfaced panels for furniture and doors. Also a plastic sheet.

Ventilation: Ventilation is the removal of contaminated air from within the building and its replacement by outdoor air. This may be done by fan equipment, opening windows, air leakage through the building envelope, or a combination of these.

Vermiculite: A magnesium, iron and silica mineral which expands when heated-forming a lightweight, fire resistant bead which is useful for insulation. The dust is hazardous to inhale.

Vitrified: A clay fired to the point of melting into a glass-like substance (glassification).

Volatile organic compounds (VOCs): Gases with organic structures (based on the carbon atom), which are emitted from materials made from polymers or containing solvents or plasticizers. Many are irritants; some are toxic.

Volatile solvents: Solvents which evaporate at room temperature, adding to indoor air pollution.

Vulcanize: Transformation of a soft or liquid rubber into a very tough, heat-resistant rubber, usually by the application of heat and sometimes the addition of sulfur. Silicone caulk vulcanizes at room temperature with little toxic emissions.

Waferboard: See Oriented strand board; Chipboard

Xylene: An aromatic component of petroleum with a sharp solvent odor. Xylene is moderately toxic and is used as a solvent for dyes, inks, paints and adhesives.

Zinc oxide: A white pigment used in paints, ointments, plastics and rubber which resists ultraviolet light and mold growth. Low toxicity, but the dust is hazardous.

RESOURCES

Books

Aberly, Doug (Ed.). *Boundaries of Home: Mapping for Local Empowerment.* Gabriola Island, BC, Philadelphia, PA: New Society Publishers, 1993.

Ashford, Nicholas, and Claudia Miller. *Chemical Exposures: Low Levels and High Stakes.* New York: Van Nostrand Reinhold, 1991.

Bower, John. *Healthy House Building: A Design and Construction Guide.* Unionville, IN: House Institute, 1993.

Brown, G.Z. *Sun, Wind and Light: Architectural Design Strategies.* New York: John Wiley and Sons, 1985.

Center for Resourceful Building Technology. *Guide to Resource Efficient Building Elements (GREBE).* PO Box 110, Missoula, MT 59806, (406) 549-7678: Center for Resourceful Building Technology, 1996. A catalog of information on resource efficient construction.

Davis, Andrew, and Paul Schaffman. *The Home Environmental Sourcebook: 50 Environmental Hazards To Avoid When Buying, Selling Or Maintaining A Home.* New York: Owl Books, Henry Holt & Co, 1996. A practical guide to home hazards.

Demkin, J., ed. *The Environmental Resource Guide.* New York: American Institute of Architects, John Wiley and Sons, 1997. An encyclopedic guide to environmental information for the design professional.

The Iris Catalog, Guide to Healthy and Iris Communications. PO Box 5920, Eugene, OR 97408-0911, (541) 484-9353. A carefully selected booklist on healthy building and energy efficiency topics.

Lstiburek, Joseph. *Builders Guide: Cold Climates.* 70 Main St., Westford, MA 01886, (508) 589-5100: Building Science Corporation. The most up-to-date book on building science for durability and moisture control in cold climates.

Spirn, Anne Whinston. *The Granite Garden: Urban Nature and Human Design.* New York: Basic Books, 1984.

Newsletters

Environmental Building News, and the *E Build Library CD ROM.* RR1 Box 161, Brattleboro, VT 05301, (802) 257-7300 [ebn@ebuild.com]. Leading information resource on healthy and environmentally responsive building.

281

Indoor Air Quality Update. Cutter Information Corp., 37 Broadway, Arlington, MA 02174-5539, (800) 964-5118. A professional, technical newsletter on indoor air quality research.

Energy Design Update. Cutter Information Corp., 37 Broadway, Arlington, MA 02174-5539, (800) 964-5118. The "industry standard" bulletin on energy efficient design and practice.

Indoor Air Bulletin, PO Box 8446, Santa Cruz, CA 95061-8446, (408) 426-6624. A thorough research and design perspective on healthy buildings and environmentally responsive practice.

Advanced Buildings Newsletter. *RAIC* (Royal Architecture Institute of Canada), 55 Murray St. Ste 330, Ottawa, ON, Canada, K1N 5M3, (613) 241-3600. An international view of environmental and high technology design and practice, emphasizing commercial buildings.

Solplan Review. The Drawing Room, Box 86627, North Vancouver, BC, Canada, V7L 4L2 Tel. / Fax. (604) 689-1841. A practical summary of recent developments in housing design, research, technology and building practice.

The Human Ecologist. Human Ecology Action League, (HEAL). PO Box 49126, Atlanta, GA 30359-1126. Newsletter, information and advocacy organization for the environmentally hypersensitive.

Interior Concerns Resource Guide. PO Box 2386, Mill Valley, CA 94942, (415) 389-8049, [www.geonetwork.org]. A listing of low toxicity building products and energy and water conserving products. Updated quarterly by subscription.

Other Resources

The Green Building Website, operated by Environmental Building News, [www.ebuild.com].

CMHC (Canada Mortgage and Housing Corp.), Canadian Housing Information Centre, 700 Montreal Rd., Ottawa, ON, Canada, K1A 0P7, (613) 748-2367.

Some Healthy Building Publications Available from CMHC

- *The Clean Air Guide*
- *Building Materials for the Environmentally Hypersensitive*
- *Housing the Environmentally Hypersensitive*
- *The Healthy Housing Design Competition*
- *The REDI Guide*. Iris Communications, PO Box 5920, Eugene, OR 97405-0911, (541) 484-9353, [www.oikos.com]. Guide to resource and energy efficient building products and information.
- Greenclips News Service Website, [www.solstice.crest.org].

Index